XX STRONG™

presents

DOMINATE YOUR PERI◊D

The #1 Educational Resource, for Female Athletes and High Achievers!

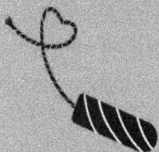

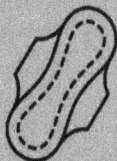

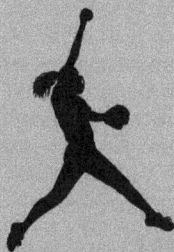

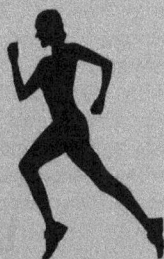

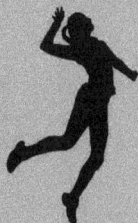

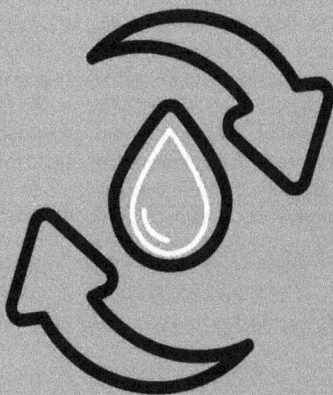

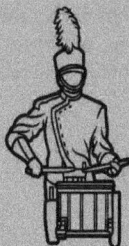

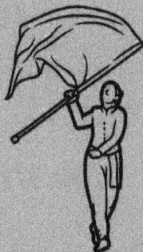

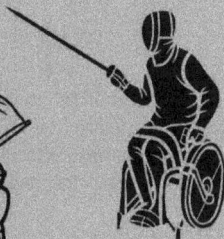

HEATHER ALLMENDINGER

with **Barb V**

HOSTS OF 2 INTERNATIOALLY TOP RATED PODCASTS

EMBRACING FLOW & **The Kid Factor**

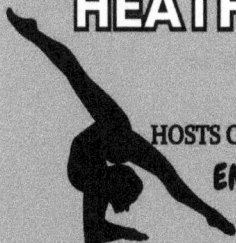

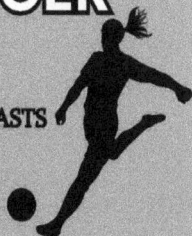

Dominate Your Period

The #1 Educational Resource for Female Athletes and High Achievers

Art and Illustrations by Heather Allmendinger and Barb V
Canva Pro graphics
Cover design and Layout by Barb V

ISBN: 979-8-89300-006-1

Published in the United States by The Kid Factor, LLC

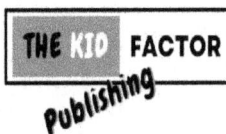

THE KID FACTOR
Publishing

PREFACE

It was the summer before fifth grade when my paternal grandmother sat me down for the dreaded 'period talk.' Little did I know that within two weeks of her well-intentioned words would mark the beginning of a three decade-long struggle. At ten years old, I was completely unprepared for the realities that awaited me.

Neither my grandmother nor the school's "period" explanation could accurately convey the agonizing cramps that would cause me to pass out on the bathroom floor, the dizzying nausea and vomiting that drove me to the nurse's office month after month, or the mortification of having to wear white sweatpants after bleeding through my dark blue pants.

For 35 years, I loathed my period, perceiving it as a cruel curse inflicted upon womankind. Even the prospect of childbearing did little to ease my resentment towards this monthly trauma. Why were women so despised, I wondered, that we had to endure such suffering?

It wasn't until I was diagnosed with precancerous cells on my cervix that my perspective began to shift. In the journey towards healing, I stumbled upon a life-altering statement:

menstrual cycles are meant to be pain-free. Skeptical yet desperate, I embarked on a protocol that promised to banish the debilitating symptoms I had long accepted as inevitable.

To my astonishment, the next cycle was my first pain-free, PMS-free, medical suppression free cycle and marked the beginning of a transformative journey – one that would lead me down a path of extensive research, training, and ultimately, the creation of this book.

Within these pages, I invite you to begin a journey of your own – a voyage that will shatter the stigma surrounding menstrual cycles and replace it with a newfound sense of empowerment and appreciation for the inherent wisdom of your body.

Together, we will unlock the secrets of four hormones that play a major role in orchestrating your cycle, equipping you with the knowledge to track your unique rhythms using a medical and science-based period awareness method. For athletes, this insight is invaluable, as disruptions in menstrual function can signal underlying issues that, left unaddressed, can derail performance, and potentially end careers.

But this book offers more than just education for those who are currently menstruating; it is a call to embrace cyclical living, aligning your mindset, habits, and lifestyle with the ever-changing ebbs and flows of your unique cycle. By attuning ourselves to our bodies' natural rhythms, we can optimize our training, recovery, performance and overall well-being.

No longer must we suffer in silence, resigning ourselves to the misguided notion that pain and discomfort are inevitable. By reclaiming our narratives and celebrating the beauty of our cycles, we can create a world where menstruation is celebrated, not stigmatized – a world where we are empowered to listen to our bodies and make informed decisions to protect our health and longevity on our chosen path.

Join me on this empowering journey and let us rewrite the narrative together – one cycle at a time, one athlete at a time, one woman at a time.

Until next time, love hard, laugh often, and always be Vivydus.

Heather M Allmendinger

PREFACE

You are the biggest and best advocate of your own health.

--- *Heather Allmendinger*

ACKNOWLEDGEMENTS:

For all those who knew they needed this information but couldn't find it and for those who didn't know they needed it.

Rachel, thank you for encouraging me when we first met to write a book about menstruation.

Megan, thank you for suggesting I speak to your friend who coaches biological female wrestlers. That planted the seed to start working with athletes and coaches.

Coach Barb V, an incredible mentor, coach, and true friend: thank you for continuously challenging me to reach new heights and for sharing in the vision of this journey. Your guidance and wisdom have enriched this book, brought the Embracing Flow podcast to life, and so much more. I am grateful for your unwavering support, your insight, and the joy of having you as a business partner.

Scott, thank you for your unconditional love and unending support through the crazy hours, ideas, and trips that brought this book and my entrepreneurial vision to life. Your steadfast belief in me has been my foundation, allowing me the freedom to pour myself into this journey. I am so grateful to share this life and mission with you.

Mason and Gunnar, thank you for your boundless love and curiosity. Though this book may not be about your world directly, you remind me daily why empowering everyone with knowledge is essential. May you grow up remembering your knowledge of this topic enhances your abilities to be better friends, partners, parents, co-workers, and leaders. I love you both.

To the incredible women of Polka Dot Powerhouse and the Renegade Unicorns, who have lifted me up along this journey. Thank you for your unwavering support, encouragement, and belief in my dreams. You've helped me think through countless ideas and processes, giving me the space to be fully myself. Your friendship and strength have been a gift, and I am so grateful to have had you by my side through this adventure.

Heather

I would like to begin by expressing my deep gratitude to Heather Allmendinger, whose incredible passion, extensive knowledge, and dedication have been instrumental in bringing this book to life. Collaborating with such a talented and driven individual has been an honor, a source of inspiration, and I look forward to our continued work together as we serve our XX Strong community of athletes and high achievers and their coaches, trainers, parents, and teams.

Reflecting on my own journey as an athlete, I realize how much I wish I had known about the role my menstrual cycle played in my performance. Despite years of training and competing at high levels, I was never taught about the impact of hormonal cycles on strength, endurance, or recovery. This missing piece of knowledge kept me from fully embracing my superpowers in ways I didn't fully understand until much later in life.

Now in menopause, I continue to experience the effects of cyclical living on my athletic performance. Learning to honor these natural rhythms has been transformative, adding new layers of understanding and respect for my body that I only wish I had discovered sooner. As I continue to train and prepare for upcoming competitions, it's my goal that through this book, we can bring greater awareness to this vital aspect of health and performance for our XX Strong athletes.

I'm immensely thankful for our publishing team, our Renegade Unicorns mastermind, the Diamond Members of Polka Dot Powerhouse and all the Chapters who have supported us and have had us speak to their members.

And to our athletes and readers, thank you for embarking on this journey with us. May these pages empower you with insights that will enrich your own life and athletic journey.

With gratitude,

Barb V

TABLE OF CONTENTS

Your period is an outward sign of your inner health!

- - - Heather Allmendinger

WELCOME TO YOUR CYCLICAL JOURNEY!

Have you ever wondered why most books treat your period as just something to deal with, like a monthly inconvenience that shows up uninvited? Well, get ready for a completely different adventure! This isn't your ordinary period book – it's your personal guide to understanding the amazing symphony of hormones that orchestrates your entire body's rhythm.

Imagine having a superpower that changes throughout the month, bringing you different strengths at different times. Guess what? You already have this power! Your menstrual cycle isn't just about your period – it's an intricate dance that affects everything from your energy levels to your creativity, from your physical capabilities to your emotional wisdom. And the best part? Once you understand this dance, you can use it to your advantage.

What makes this book different? While other books might tell you about tracking your period or dealing with symptoms, we're diving into how your whole body works together in perfect harmony. Your hormones aren't just doing one job – they're like air traffic controllers, coordinating everything from your brain to your muscles, your energy to your emotions.

But here's where this is really different: we're combining cutting-edge science with ancient wisdom and modern technology. You'll discover how your cycle connects with the phases of the moon, learn about a revolutionary technique called The F.I.X. Code, a Non-Invasive Guided Quantum Visualization, and find out how to work with your body instead of against it.

Think of this book as your personal laboratory, diary, and guide all rolled into one. You'll find:

- Scientific explanations that actually make sense (no boring textbook talk here!)
- Fun activities that help you understand your unique rhythm
- Tracking tools that reveal patterns you never knew existed
- Natural alternatives to traditional solutions
- Mind-body techniques that tap into your brain's incredible power
- Ways to connect with the natural cycles around you

This isn't just about tracking your period – it's about discovering how your cycle influences your entire life. Want to know when you might have the most energy for sports or doing a presentation? Curious about why you feel super creative some weeks and more focused others? Interested in understanding how your hormones affect your study/work habits? We've got you covered!

For too long, we've been taught to view our cycles as something to overcome or ignore. But what if your cycle is your secret weapon? What if understanding these natural rhythms could help you excel in school, sports, work, relationships, and life? That's exactly what we're here to explore together.

Whether you're just starting your menstrual journey, or you've been cycling for years, this book meets you where you are. It's written for anyone aged 12 and up who wants to understand their body better and harness its natural power. You'll find information about important topics like relative energy deficiency (RED-S), period awareness, and various options for managing common cycle – all explained in a way that's easy to understand and actually fun to learn about.

Ready to transform how you think about your cycle? Ready to discover the power that's been within you all along? Then turn the page – your journey to understanding, embracing, and celebrating your cyclical nature starts now. Welcome to a new way of living that's perfectly in tune with your body's natural rhythm!

Before we dive in, let's take a moment to capture your current thoughts about your cycle. On the next page, you'll find a "My Cycle Perspective" worksheet. Don't worry about having the "right" answers – this is just for you to track your journey. At the end of the book, you'll fill out a similar page, and you might be amazed at how differently you see things! After all, knowledge is power, and you're about to become very powerful indeed.

Let's begin this adventure together – because understanding your cycle isn't just about marking days on a calendar. It's about unlocking a whole new way of living that celebrates the incredible wisdom of your body.

Heather M. Allmendinger, CHC, MBA

Certified Heath Coach, Masters
Business Administration
Fertility Awareness Instructor

WELCOME TO YOUR CYCLICAL JOURNEY!

My Cycle Perspective: Before Our Journey

Date: _____

How I Currently View My Cycle

- What three words come to mind when you think about your cycle?

    1. _____

    2. _____

    3. _____

Current Pros & Cons of My Cycle

Pros (What I Like/Appreciate):

    1. _____

    2. _____

    3. _____

Cons (What I Find Challenging):

    1. _____

    2. _____

    3. _____

WELCOME TO YOUR CYCLICAL JOURNEY!

Quick Questions:

- How much do you feel you understand about your cycle?

  (Circle one)

  > Not at all - A little - Somewhat - Pretty well - Very well

- How connected do you feel to your cycle? (Circle one)

  > Not at all - A little - Somewhat - Very - Extremely

- What do you hope to learn from this book?

  _____

  _____

  _____

  _____

  _____

- NOTES:

  _____

  _____

  _____

  _____

  _____

THE F.I.X. CODE

In early November 2024 I participated as a contestant in the Ms. division of the United States of America's Miss Pennsylvania 2025 Pageant. I chose this organization because of its inclusivity and its mission to Empower Women, Inspire Others, and Uplift Everyone. It had been 27 years since my last pageant, so going into pageant weekend I was comfortable yet as pageant day arrived had an unsettled feeling inside me. I remembered the interview round at my last pageant, and I did well, however didn't have answers to some of the questions and I was afraid history would repeat itself. I tried my go-to grounding exercises and they helped settle the nerves a little, but not where I felt solid and in my power. I was very prepared to compete, even against the beautiful ladies in my division that had been continuously doing pageants for many years.

It was finally my group's turn to enter the round robin interview room. We had three minutes with four judges. Overall, the interviews went well, I knew I could have done better, however overall I was pleased with my performance, yet still had that unsettled feeling in my gut.

Between interviews and show time we had rehearsals and some down time. I did more grounding exercises, breathing exercises, visualizations, all the tools given to me that had worked in the past. As the afternoon turned into evening, I started feeling more and more in my power, the show started, I was a shining star on stage, walked with high energy and confidently on stage in a bikini with a middle-aged mom body, elegantly presented myself in evening wear, and then it came time for the anxiety inducing on-stage surprise question. Each division was asked a unique question, and only the contestant on stage knew what the question was. The other contestants waited backstage wearing noise-canceling earplugs so they couldn't hear. As I awaited my turn to adorn the stage in my beautiful, sparkly gown, I had a very uneasy feeling in my gut that I just couldn't remove. It kept growing the closer it got to my turn on stage. I again tried breathing exercises, shaking it off, visualization, all the tools I had that worked for me in the past, it didn't dispel the feeling. As my turn approached, I walked up the backstage steps, removed my earplugs, and gracefully walked on stage. Smiled at the judges, made a quick smile look around the auditorium, and then greeted the emcee. He gave the on-stage question's instructions, read the question twice, and tilted the microphone towards me to answer. The question had two parts, one about my platform and the second part of how it fits within the mission of the organization. This question in some form, I had been answering for months and could answer in my sleep. It was what some would call a beachball question, it really couldn't have been much easier. Yet, at this particular point in time, I froze, my mind went blank. I looked at the judges, opened my mouth, words feverishly poured out, as I finished my answer, I gave a look around the auditorium, said thank you and then saw the confused look on the emcee's face. At that precise moment, I realized I had only answered half the question and my chances of coming home with a high placement or even the crown was gone.

I spent that night and the next two weeks fixated on how I messed up that question, and how I could have answered it better. I spoke to my dear friend Barb the next day and she said, "you needed a F.I.X. Code session, why didn't you call me?"! Well, I had done several sessions with her in the past, yet for some reason, I didn't think what I was doing applied. Boy, was I wrong in that thought process. The F.I.X. Code can be used in almost any situation. Had I used it earlier that day or even while waiting for my turn, the outcome could have been completely different.

What is The F.I.X. Code? The F.I.X. Code is a Non-Invasive Guided Quantum Visualization technique - a groundbreaking approach in athletics, competition, and personal growth rooted and backed by neuroscience.

This method works by leveraging the brain's neuroplasticity - its ability to form new neural connections throughout life. With the guidance and assistance of your Master Certified F.I.X. Code Method Coach, mine is my friend Barb V, here's how becoming a F.I.X.ed athlete or high achiever can benefit you:

- **Rewire your brain:** Science shows that repeated thoughts and experiences strengthen neural pathways. This technique helps eliminate negative pathways while reinforcing positive ones.

- **Harness your subconscious:** Research indicates that up to 95% of our brain activity occurs at the subconscious level. By addressing subconscious blocks, this method assists in creating profound change.

- **Align your conscious and unconscious mind:** Studies reveal that conflicting beliefs between our conscious and unconscious minds can hinder our progress. This technique helps bring these into harmony and balance.

The F.I.X. Code allows you to:

- Disconnect negative emotions from past memories

- Reduce and potentially eliminate future anxieties, worries, fears, and feelings that hold you back

- Cultivate a more positive outlook

By addressing emotional experiences stored in your subconscious and unconscious mind, you can overcome barriers holding you back from attaining joy, success, and fulfillment.

Whether you're a driven athlete, coach, personal trainer, a business professional, a dedicated parent, or an ambitious youth, this science-based training tool offers a path to living 'on-point' - fully present and engaged in every moment and focused on every performance.

Experience the transformative power of The F.I.X. Code and embark on your journey as a more empowered, vibrant athlete by booking your free 15-minute introductory session now. No strings attached, no sales pitch, just you harnessing the full power and benefit of The F.I.X. Code with Barb V or one of our Internationally Certified F.I.X. Code Coaches.

Become A F.I.X.ed Athlete

Elevate your athletic performance with The F.I.X. Code, this non-Invasive quantum guided visualization - is a cutting-edge mental training technology for athletes at every level.

Scientifically grounded, this approach taps into the power of your mind to enhance your physical and mental performances. Here's how it can transform your performances:

- **Mental resilience:** Strengthen neural pathways associated with focus, determination, and grit. Whether you're a weekend warrior, a pro athlete, or kicking butt in the board room; this technique helps you dominate mental barriers.

- **Overcome performance anxiety:** By addressing subconscious fears and past setbacks, you can perform with newfound confidence. Visualize success and disconnect from negative emotions that may be holding you back. Ending slumps quickly and effortlessly.

- **Faster recovery:** Harness the mind-body connection to potentially speed up your body's healing and reduce recovery time. Studies show that positive visualization can influence physical healing processes.

The F.I.X. Code allows athletes and high achievers to:

- Let go of past failures or injuries that may be impacting current performances

- Reduce pre-game jitters and performance anxiety

- Eliminate negative self-talk

- Generate athletic and personal gains in and out of competitions

- Develop a champion's mindset for peak performance

By aligning your conscious goals with your subconscious mind, you will unlock your fullest potential. The F.I.X. Code addresses the emotional experiences and future worries that might be blocking your path to excellence.

Whether you're a young athlete dreaming of going pro, a college player aiming for the big leagues, or a seasoned professional looking to stay at the top of your game, The F.I.X. Code offers a way to perform at your absolute best.

Ready to take your mental game to the next level? Experience the game-changing effects of The F.I.X. Code and unleash your inner champion. It's time to perform on-point, every time you step onto the field, court, track, or into the board room! Reach out to Barb and her team today at www.BarbV.Fun

Quantum Field Goal Setting:

A Guide for Athletes and High Achievers Harnessing their Power of Intention

Imagine you're about to take a crucial shot in basketball, you're at the starting line of a race, or about to give a presentation to a CEO or mega client. Now, what if I told you that your thoughts and intentions at that moment could influence the outcome, not just through your actions, but at a fundamental level of reality? This is the essence of Quantum Field Goal Setting.

The Basics

- **Everything is Energy:** At the most basic level, everything in the universe - including you and your thoughts - is made up of energy and vibrations.

- **The Observer Effect:** In quantum physics, there's a principle called the observer effect. It suggests that the mere act of observing a particle can change its behavior.

- **You are the Observer:** As an athlete or high achiever, you're not just a passive participant in your performance. You're an active observer and influencer of your reality.

How It Works

- **Setting the Intention:** Instead of just thinking about your goal, you're going to set an intention at your deepest level. This means fully immersing yourself in the vision and certainty of achieving your goal.

- **Aligning Your Energy:** Through focused mindfulness and visualization, you align your body's energy with the frequency of your goal. It's like tuning a radio to the exact station you want.

- **Collapsing Possibilities:** In quantum physics, particles exist in multiple states until observed. Similarly, your potential outcomes exist in multiple states until you focus your total intention.

Practical Steps

- **Clarity:** Define your goal with crystal clarity. Instead of "I want to win," specify "I will score the winning point in the final 10 seconds." or "I will have a signed contract before I leave this customers office."

- **Emotional Engagement:** Feel the positive emotions of achieving this goal. Experience the joy, the rush, the sense of accomplishment as if it's happening now.

- **Quantum Mindfulness:** Invest 10-15 minutes daily in deep focus; visualizing your goal as already accomplished. See every detail, activate every one of your senses, feel every positive sensation. Live and breathe your goal with all that you are.

- **Physical Anchoring:** Create a powerful physical gesture (like touching your heart) that instantly connects you to this total state of achievement. Use it before, during, and throughout your practices, performances, and day.

- **Detachment:** Paradoxically, after setting your intention, detach from the outcome. Trust that the quantum field is aligning to your intentions and energies.

The Science Behind It

While it might sound mystical, there's emerging science supporting this approach:

- **Studies on heart-brain coherence** show that our hearts generate a powerful electromagnetic field that can affect our surroundings.

- **Research on the placebo effect** demonstrates the power of belief in creating physical changes in the body.

- **Experiments in quantum physics**, like the double-slit experiment, suggest that consciousness can influence the behavior of particles.

For the High School Athlete

Think of it like this: You're not just training your body; you're training reality itself to match your goals. Every time you practice Quantum Field Goal Setting, you're sending out a powerful signal to the universe about what you intend to achieve. Like the science behind the technology of your cell phone and sending and receiving direct messages; you have the same power within your conscious and subconscious mind to send and receive those direct messages of your intentions and goals.

Many athletes do not get this type of information and training until they reach the upper levels of elite status in their sport. Learning, training, and working with a qualified and certified F.I.X. Code Coach at this stage of your athletic journey will only exponentially enhance your athletic and life performances.

For the Professional

The F.I.X. Code can give you an edge when physical training has reached its peak. It's about optimizing the unseen aspects of performance - your energy field, your subconscious beliefs, and even the quantum field around you. Use this to break through any plateaus and achieve seemingly impossible feats.

Know that this isn't about magical thinking. It's about aligning every aspect of your being - from your thoughts to your cellular energy - with your goals. Your body and brain are constantly communicating, creating pathways that influence how you feel and function throughout your cycle. The F.I.X. Code taps into this incredible mind-body connection, using your brain's natural ability to create new neural pathways. Think of it like installing new software that helps your computer run better - except in this case, you're helping your brain to better understand and work with your body's natural rhythms.

As you'll discover in the next chapter, your menstrual cycle involves complex hormonal changes that affect your entire body. By using The F.I.X. Code technology, you can enhance your awareness of these changes and even influence how you experience them. Just as athletes use visualization to improve their performance, you can use The F.I.X. Code to better understand and work with your cycle's natural ebbs and flows. This isn't about forcing changes - it's about creating a deeper connection between your unconscious and conscious mind and body, allowing them to work together in harmony with your natural rhythms. We'll discuss how this is done later in the book.

So, are you wondering what happened, where did I place? As I had known, I failed to place in the Top 3. I was 3rd Runner Up or placed 4th in my division, however my performance from enrollment through pageant weekend earned me the highest award possible outside of winning the crown. It is known as the Director's Award or the Empower, Inspire, Uplift award. This award is given to the state delegate who embodies the mission of the organization to Empower Women, Inspire Others, and Uplift Everyone. To me this is a huge win!

Follow me on social media, for the rest of the story and how I embraced The F.I.X. Code to enhance my future performances…

- What is The F.I.X. Code
- How to become a F.I.X.ed individual
- Importance of visualization and mindset
- How The F.I.X. Code is different from other methods

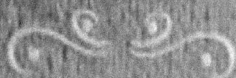

UNITED STATES
OF AMERICA'S
MISS PENNSYLVANIA
2025

Empower Inspire Uplift

THE MENSTRUAL CYCLE

First, what is a menstrual cycle? It is a natural monthly hormonal routine the XX chromosome (biological female) body uses to maintain the overall health of 11 bodily systems using the rise and fall of specific hormones ending in a shedding of the endometrial lining. This monthly cycle starts around the average age of 12 and ends naturally around the average age of 54. This type of menstrual cycle is unique to only a handful of mammals including humans, two families of monkeys, chimpanzees, the elephant shrew, bats, and a spiny mouse. Other mammals have estrous ('estrəs) cycles where the biological female animal goes through a similar process however absorbs the endometrial lining, the exception to this is dogs.

Menstrual cycles are unique to each individual and come in many lengths. From menarche (first period) through menopause (12 months after last period), your unique cycle can and will change its average length several times. A cycle length is calculated by counting the number of days from the first day of red bleeding through the day before the bleeding begins again. Another way to explain this is that cycle day 1 is the first day of steady red blood.

The final day of that cycle is the day before steady red blood is seen again. In between these days of red blood are days without bleeding and days with possible brown, black, or pink blood. Blood of all colors means different things, most of the time blood seen during the cycle are signs of hormonal misalignment. We'll go into more detail on tracking and possible causes a little later in this book.

Although they come in many lengths, cycles can be grouped into three categories; short, standard, and long. Short cycles are under 24 days, standard cycles are 24-36 days, and long cycles are over 36 days. A regular cycle arrives within a 6-day range of your unique average cycle length (ex. Month 1 is 28 days, month 2 is 30 days, and month 3 is 26 days), an irregular cycle is outside 6 days from the previous cycle or average, (ex. Month 1 is 36 days, month 2 is 45 days, and month 3 is 28 days). An average cycle length is 28/29 days amongst those in their reproductive years (average ages 14-42), similar to the moon/lunar cycle that is 28 days. It's typical for menstrual cycles to take 12-24 months to regulate and become consistent after the first period. However, if cycles remain irregular,

THE MENSTRUAL CYCLE

excessively heavy, or painful after 24 months from the first menstruation, it's advisable to seek medical attention. Additionally, if your luteal phase (the phase after ovulation) lasts fewer than 9 days, or if you experience anovulatory cycles (meaning no ovulation occurs) and you aren't taking medication that stops ovulation, it's recommended to consult a healthcare professional. These patterns may indicate a hormonal dysfunction, which, if left unaddressed, can lead to serious health issues in your 20s and beyond. Similarly, if you're between 21 and 37 years old and experience more than three atypical to you cycles in a 12-month

> "Just as abnormal blood pressure, heart rate, or respiratory rate may be key to diagnosis of potentially serious health conditions, identification of abnormal menstrual patterns through adolescence may permit early identification of potential health concerns for adulthood."
> --- AAP and ACOG

period, or if you have two consecutive atypical cycles to you lasting under 24 days or over 36 days, it could be a sign of an underlying hormonal issue.

The American Academy of Pediatrics and The American College of Obstetrics and Gynecology note that a menstrual cycle is

THE MENSTRUAL CYCLE

a vital sign for adolescents, "Just as abnormal blood pressure, heart rate, or respiratory rate may be key to diagnosis of potentially serious health conditions, identification of abnormal menstrual patterns through adolescence may permit early identification of potential health concerns for adulthood."

When visiting your doctor, they will ask you the date of your last menstrual period (LMP) and some may ask the length of your cycle, how many days you bleed, and how many product changes you perform in a day during menstruation. These are important to know so your doctor can determine what hormone testing could be needed or what might be happening inside your body. The overall health of your body communicates with you through your menstrual cycle. It is a doctor's visit every single month.

This book is also a good resource to take with you as it will show how your cycle is functioning through all phases, if tracking is followed as instructed. Our periods are outward signs of inner health. They are a vital sign and share valuable information. So how does our body cause this cycle to work? I'm so glad you

THE MENSTRUAL CYCLE

asked, through chemical messengers called hormones.

Summary:

- Menstrual cycles are a natural and healthy body function
- An average cycle is 28 days, cycles can come in various length and still be considered healthy
- Humans are one of only a few species that experience monthly bleeding
- Menstrual cycles are outward signs of inner health

The overall health of your body communicates with you through your menstrual cycle. It is a doctor's visit every single month.

HORMONES – YOUR BODY'S MESSENGERS

Our bodies communicate between the 11 bodily systems using hormones, also known as chemical messengers. These messengers tell our bodies how to operate and grow. There are over 50 known hormones in the human body with 12 of these hormones directly involved in the menstrual cycle and other bodily functions. Because the menstrual cycle incorporates almost 20% of the known hormones, it is easy to see how a period is seen as an outward sign of inner health.

Although there are 12 hormones directly involved with each cycle, to keep things simple, we will only be discussing four of the cycle hormones in this book, follicular stimulating hormone, estrogen, luteinizing hormone, and progesterone. The remaining eight hormones will be discussed and incorporated with these four in a future book.

The hormone to kick off puberty and each cycle is the follicular stimulating hormone (FSH). It is produced in the pituitary gland located in the brain. In puberty, FSH triggers the ovaries to increase estrogen which helps with breast development and menstruation. During the reproductive years FSH is used to regulate the menstrual cycle. It is released right before or a day or two into menstruation to stimulate several ovarian follicles (a tiny fluid filled sac in the ovaries that has the potential to develop an ovum) to wake up and begin growing, starting the monthly hormonal cycle each month. Once FSH peaks it decreases to pre-menstruation levels, the decrease to pre-menstrual levels triggers the ovaries to produce heavy hitter estrogen.

Estrogen is considered a growth hormone, it is primarily produced and regulated in the ovaries during the reproductive years. Before puberty and after menopause estrogen is produced in the adrenal glands (small glands above the kidneys) and adipose tissue (body fat). Estrogen helps grow ovarian follicles, mature an ovarian follicle ovum, increases the endometrial (uterine) lining, activates the pituitary gland to release luteinizing hormone for ovulation, contracts the uterus, grows breast tissue, helps form bones, makes blood vessels bigger, stops blood from flowing, strengthens brain activity, and keeps moods balanced. High levels of estrogen in relation to progesterone can cause anxiety around the end of each monthly menstrual cycle and high estrogen levels is linked to endometriosis, breast cancer, and a multitude of other cancers and health issues. See why I call this hormone a heavy hitter, it is a necessary hormone for proper body function, yet can be damaging if unchecked. Once this slugger hits it's peak around ovulation, the brain releases the sister to FSH, luteinizing hormone. Estrogen then decreases slightly, yet stays elevated for the remainder of the cycle until a few days before menstruation begins.

Luteinizing Hormone (LH) is produced in the brain by the pituitary gland. It is a very close hormone to FSH, although does a different job. LH is triggered by high levels of estrogen in the ovaries as ovarian follicles mature. When ovarian follicle(s) mature the brain signals a release of LH. The released LH tells the ovarian follicle with the most mature ovum to open and spit out the ovum into the fallopian tubes, known as ovulation. Once the ovum is released, LH is used to develop a new temporary gland in the now vacant ovarian follicle every month called the corpus luteum. This new organ produces progesterone, our feel good, chill hormone. Once ovulation occurs, LH returns to pre-ovulation levels.

Progesterone is made in the ovaries by the corpus luteum, a temporary gland that is made each month during the reproductive years after ovulation takes place. Once in menopause or when using hormonal birth control, progesterone is produced in the adrenal glands in a significantly smaller quantity. Progesterone is considered a stabilizing and calming hormone. Progesterone's role is to relax the uterine muscles, stop the endometrial lining growth from ovulation until menstruation, slows or stops the growth of breast tissue, maintains bone health, releases the built up of fluids in the body (water retention), helps us to have bowel movements, heals

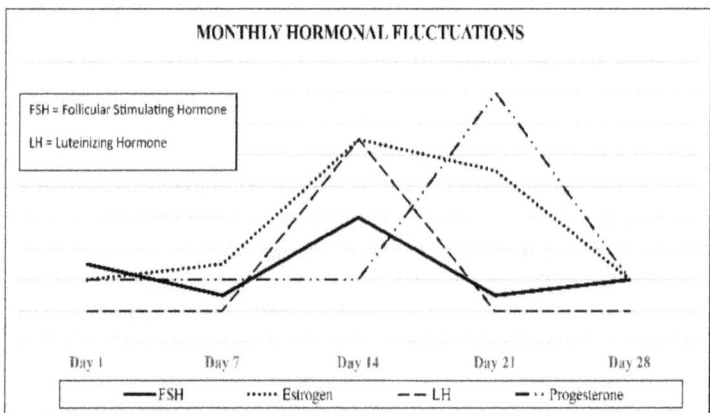

MONTHLY HORMONAL FLUCTUATIONS

FSH = Follicular Stimulating Hormone
LH = Luteinizing Hormone

Day 1   Day 7   Day 14   Day 21   Day 28

——— FSH   ······ Estrogen   — — LH   — ·· Progesterone

HORMONES – YOUR BODY'S MESSENGERS

brain cells, promotes better quality sleep, enables relaxation, and if pregnancy occurs, holds onto the uterine lining until labor begins. High levels of progesterone in relation to estrogen are linked to feelings of depression around the end of each monthly menstrual cycle.

As mentioned before these are only four of the twelve hormones involved in the very intricate symphony of the menstrual cycle and your period. Many things can disrupt this symphony like medication, stress, poor nutrition, excessive exercise, illness, sleep deprivation, all leading to symptoms of hormonal alignment issues like missed periods, irregular cycles, hot flashes, breast tenderness, weak or brittle bones, trouble concentrating, headaches, feeling tired, trouble sleeping, mood changes, and many more. There are over 200 different indications of premenstrual syndrome (PMS), a combination of physical and emotional symptoms that appear from three to ten days before a period arrives and PMS's big sister Premenstrual Dysphoric Disorder (PMDD). Some may find temporary relief from these conditions by using hormonal birth control. There are other options, and they will be discussed in a little bit when we dive deeper into each phase of the menstrual cycle. Before we go there though, let's learn a little more about how these hormones work in symphony with our entire bodies.

Summary:

- The body regulates over 50 hormones in the body, 12 are directly involved with menstruation
- The pituitary gland produces and regulates the follicular stimulating hormone and luteinizing hormone
- The ovaries produce and regulate estrogen and progesterone

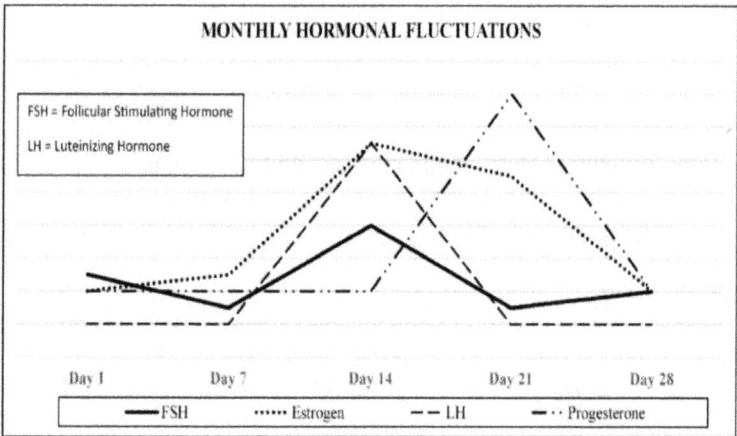

MONTHLY HORMONAL FLUCTUATIONS

FSH = Follicular Stimulating Hormone
LH = Luteinizing Hormone

Day 1   Day 7   Day 14   Day 21   Day 28

———FSH   ······ Estrogen   — — LH   — ·· Progesterone

HORMONES – YOUR BODY'S MESSENGERS

46

THE BIOLOGICAL FEMALE BODY

Our bodies are outstanding machines, each part has a purpose and important function for the machine to work in harmony. The reproductive system, home of our periods, is just a single system in the body, yet it is connected to the other ten systems using those hormones we just spoke about. If you remember, we spoke about heavy hitter estrogen, this hormone is found in every cell in our body spurring action and plays a role in all our body systems. It's teammate progesterone calms estrogen's actions when in alignment. These two hormones are used directly or indirectly by all 11 body systems: circulatory system (cardiovascular or heart), central nervous system (brain and spinal cord), endocrine system (metabolism), gastrointestinal system (digestion), immune system (illness), lymphatic system (drainage), respiratory system (breathing), integumentary system (skin, hair, nails), urinary system (waste removal), musculoskeletal system (bones, muscles, tendons, etc.), and reproductive system.

When you look at the chart on the next page, can you see how each hormone interacts with the 11 bodily systems? It's why it will be repeated many times that periods are vital and an outward sign of inner health. They are more than just for reproduction or having children. They are a doctor's visit every month.

HORMONE	DESCRIPTION	WHEN IS IT ACTIVE	WHAT DOES IT DO
Follicular Stimulating Hormone	• Produced by and released from the pituitary gland in the brain.	• From late luteal through beginning of follicular	• Regulates the cycle • Begins the development of ovarian follicles
Estrogen	• Produced and released in the ovaries • Growth hormone • Big player in menstrual cycle	• Begins activity a few days into menstruation, hits peak at ovulation, drops some after ovulation, and drops to low levels right before menstruation	• Grows and matures ovarian follicles • Tones and contracts the uterus • Enlarges the endometrial lining • Boosts breast tissue • Replenishes bone • Increases blood flow • Improves blood clotting • Elevates blood sugar • Causes fluid retention (bloating) • Stimulates brain cells • At normal levels it promotes healthy wellbeing, at high levels increases anxiety
Luteinizing Hormone	• Produced by and released from the pituitary gland in the brain.	• Ovulation	• Causes a mature ovarian follicle to rupture and release the ovum into the fallopian tubes, also known as ovulation
Progesterone	• Produced in the ovaries after ovulation • Is used to create a new organ called the Corpus Luteum each month	• From ovulation through the end of the cycle	• Feel good calming hormone • Relaxes the uterus • Holds the endometrial lining • Reduces breast tissue to your base level • Maintains bone health • Shrinks blood vessels to typical size • Lessens blood clotting • Lessens blood sugar levels • Releases excess water • Maintains and heals brain cells • Promotes sleep and relaxation; decreases anxiety, could increase depression

Our bodies need the reproduction system just as much as the other systems, yet we tend to treat it like it's able to be thrown away. Or the reproductive body parts are dirty to speak of, so we try and cover up uncomfortable conversation with different more socially acceptable names. My question to you, would you call a heart something other than a heart, an eye something other than an eye or a hand something other than a hand? No.

Yet, the reproductive system parts have been assigned many "cute" names and sometimes these names become interchangeable when they are actually completely different body parts. To get a little more comfortable with the names and locations, within this chapter there is a diagram with the female reproductive parts including the correct names and what each part does within our body. Knowing the proper names will help you communicate more efficiently with parents, partners, children, and medical professionals over the course of your life. When using the correct body part names while raising children, it will also help them communicate better with you so you know when medical attention or other services are needed. Why is this? Great question.

By using accurate language, you empower yourself to communicate clearly about your health, ensuring you receive appropriate care, and take ownership of your body. Remember, there's no shame in using correct anatomical terms – they're not just for medical textbooks, but for everyday life too.

I share the story of a mom who taught her daughter to call her vulva a "cookie" because vulva is taboo and uncomfortable to

THE BIOLOGICAL FEMALE BODY

say. The daughter went to elementary school and told the teacher that her uncle touched her "cookie". The teacher responded with praise on sharing her cookie with the uncle. What the teacher failed to understand was the young girl had been referring to her vulva instead of a food item. This young girl was brave enough to say something terrible was happening to her, however the teacher didn't understand the communication because the young girl was taught to call her vulva a cookie.

Another example: Imagine visiting your doctor with concerns about a rash "down there." The doctor asks some clarifying questions on where down there and you are unable to describe where, leading to additional embarrassing questions. After some confusion and mortifying embarrassment, you're able to clarify that the rash is on your vulva. This situation, though awkward, highlights why using proper terms for body parts is crucial. "Vulva" precisely identifies the external biological female genitalia, while vague terms like "down there" or cutesy nicknames could be in reference to legs or general pubic region. By using accurate language, you empower yourself to communicate clearly about your health, ensuring you receive appropriate care, and **take ownership** of **your** body.

Remember, there's no shame in using correct anatomical terms –

they're not just for medical textbooks, but for everyday life too.

Summary:

- The human body is an amazing machine
- Reproductive hormones impact every bodily system
- Using correct anatomical names empowers you to take ownership of your body

BIOLOGICAL FEMALE REPRODUCTIVE SYSTEM

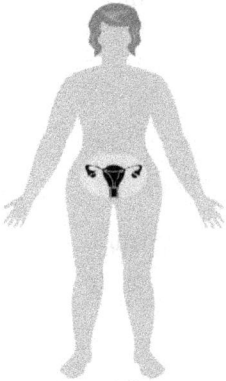

Front View

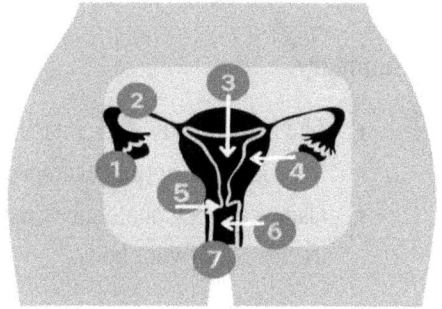

Enlarged Front View

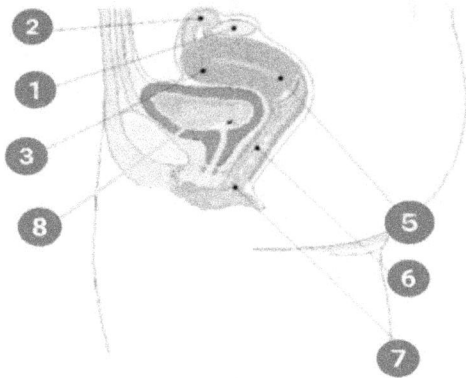

Side View

NUMBER	NAME	ROLE
1	Ovary	A pair of oval sacs that hold all ovarian follicles prior to ovulation. Also generates the corpus luteum after ovulation.
2	Fallopian Tube	A pair of tubes that carries an egg (ovum) from the ovary to the uterus
3	Uterus/Womb	Strong upside-down pear-shaped organ used to carry and grow a baby or babies
4	Endometrial lining	Lining of the uterus that grows during the follicular phase and sheds at menstruation. This is also the place where an embryo attaches itself for nutrients during pregnancy.
5	Cervix	The cervix is a muscular canal that links the uterus to the vagina. This organ allows for the passage of fluids between the uterine and vaginal cavities. It plays a vital role in the cycling of menstrual flow and the birth process itself.
6	Vagina	Is a muscular, hollow tube that extends from the vaginal opening to the cervix. The vagina's muscular walls are lined with mucous membranes, which keep it protected and moist.
7	Vulva	The external part of the female reproductive system. Located between the legs, the vulva covers the opening to the vagina and other reproductive organs inside the body.
8	Bladder	A sac that holds urine until released when using the restroom.

THE BIOLOGICAL FEMALE BODY

By using accurate language, you empower yourself to communicate clearly about your health, ensuring you receive appropriate care, and take ownership of your body. Remember, there's no shame in using correct anatomical terms – they're not just for medical textbooks, but for everyday life too.

MENSTRUAL CYCLE PHASES

So now that we know about these four hormones and how they play a role in our cycles, did you know that the cycle has phases and each hormone has a spotlight during each phase?

FSH, estrogen, LH, and progesterone have major rolls at different times during the menstrual cycle. Your cycle has two halves that break down into four phases; menstruation, follicular, ovulation, and luteal.

The first half is called the follicular phase. The follicular phase begins on Cycle Day 1 of your period and lasts until the day of ovulation. It can vary in length due to stress, illness, medications, excessive exercise, poor nutrition, among many other factors.

The length of the follicular phase determines the length of your cycle for that month. There is a lot of hormonal activity that happens during this half. The follicular phase is broken into three sections, menstruation, follicular, and ovulation. FSH, estrogen, and LH take the spotlight in these sections.

1	2	3	4	5	6	7	8	9	10	11	12	13	14	15	16	17	18	19	20	21	22	23	24	25	26	27	28

MENSTRUATION   **FOLLICULAR**   **LUTEAL**

OVULATION

MONTHLY HORMONAL FLUCTUATIONS

FSH = Follicular Stimulating Hormone

LH = Luteinizing Hormone

Day 1   Day 7   Day 14   Day 21   Day 28

———FSH   ······ Estrogen   – – LH   — ·· Progesterone

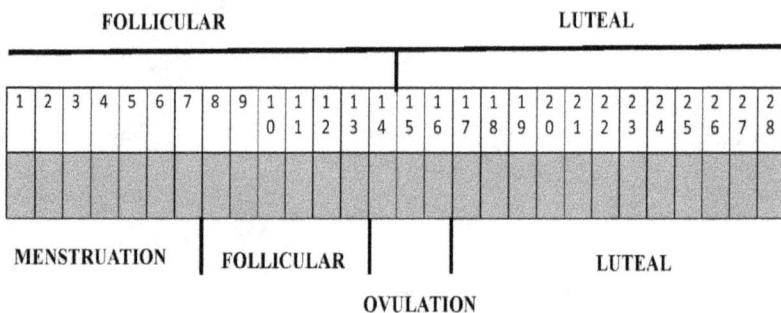

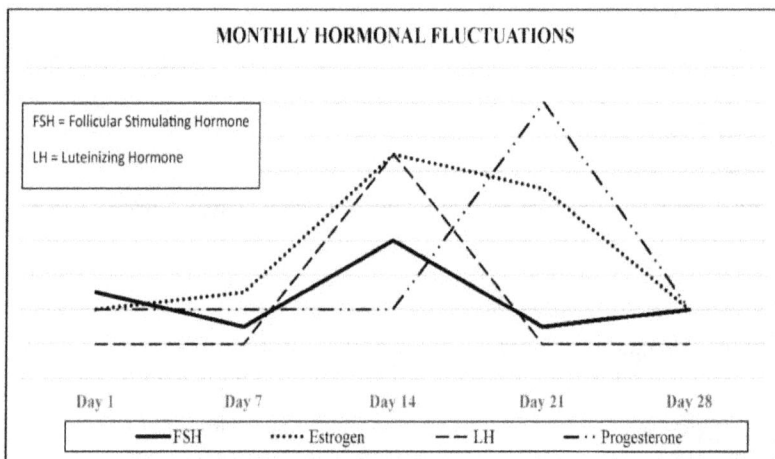

The second half is the Luteal phase. This phase begins on the day following ovulation and continues until the day before the next menstrual period starts. In a typical healthy cycle, the luteal phase lasts between 9 to 18 days, with an average duration of 12 days. Notably, the length of this phase remains consistent across your menstrual cycles, serving as a reflection of the overall hormonal activity during that cycle. The beautiful thing about this phase, once you learn your pattern, you'll know when you ovulated, then you know how many days until your period will arrive. Several days before your period arrives, there is a rapid decrease of progesterone and estrogen and rising FSH. This fluctuation in hormones is kicking off the first phase of the cycle menstruation.

MENSTRUATION:

Thought For This Phase: *My body is shedding what is no longer needed, making way for renewal. I honor this natural cycle with gentleness and self-care. I am in tune with my body's rhythms and embrace this time of release and restoration.*

The cycle begins with menstruation or bleeding. During menstruation, your body is releasing a lot of what it doesn't need and is really, really low in energy. One may find this to be a painful time in their cycle. The pain some feel is from the uterus squeezing itself tightly to help release the endometrial lining. Some ways to reduce or remove the pain is through warm washcloths across the lower belly, warm baths, showers, pain medication, or eating foods

MENSTRUAL CYCLE PHASES

high in Omega 3 fatty acids, magnesium, and B-Complex vitamins the week or two leading up to menstruation. It is the lowest energy portion in the cycle. Progesterone and estrogen are both at their lowest points at the same time during this phase. The low levels of progesterone and estrogen trigger the pituitary gland to deploy FSH. FSH tells your ovaries to begin choosing which developing follicles will begin the maturing process.

The length of bleeding can vary each cycle due to hormonal fluctuations. Healthful hormonal levels are seen by having an average 3-7 days of menstruation with at least one or two days of medium (3 to 4 product changes per day) to heavy (a product change within an hour, 5+ product changes per day, or an overnight product change) bleeding. Typical menstruation releases 40 - 80 ml (8 - 16 teaspoons) of blood over the course of a single period. A light period would involve losing less than 40 ml (less than 8 teaspoons) and a heavy period would involve losing more than 80 ml (over 16 teaspoons). Note: endometrial lining, clots, & mucus add volume to

MENSTRUAL CYCLE PHASES

menstrual flow. This is why it appears to be much more than a few teaspoons of fluid.

Menstruation is designed to be almost to completely pain-free with minimal heavy flow, and clots under the size of a dime. If you are experiencing heavy, painful, nauseating menstrual flow, this is a good indication that your hormonal levels are out of alignment or insufficient. This IS your body telling you something is out of alignment.

Menstruation is a great time to rest, read, take naps, visualize, and relax. Rest and relaxation during this section fuels the high energy of the next two sections, follicular and ovulation. For those high achievers who's schedules are booked from wake up to bed, during this phase, schedule time to rest. I know it is challenging and feels counterproductive, however the rest is needed. I work with executive level business women and suggest to them during menstruation to let the body know it will rest once the necessary work is complete or do the absolutely necessary tasks of the day and rest. There will be plenty of time and energy to finish tasks. I give

MENSTRUAL CYCLE PHASES

this example to a high achiever that teaches classes. Look at your schedule, let your body know you have 3 classes at two hours a piece that you must teach. When these classes are over honor and give gratitude to your body by going home and resting the remainder of that evening. Our bodies are cyclical and scheduling rest can be incorporated into our month. Delegate some responsibilities for a day or two. By taking it easy and being kind to your body for at least a day or two will definitely help set you up with more energy in a few days, allowing you the opportunity to hit a new record, achieve a goal, increase work productivity, and significantly reduce burnout. Foods to help support the body during this phase include beets, buckwheat, watermelon, shellfish, duck, ham, and cranberries.

HYGIENE PRODUCTS

When menstruation happens, there are many different styles and types of hygiene products available to protect clothing and allow us to go about our daily lives. Some products are disposable where others are reusable, some can be worn outside the body while others are inserted into the body to absorb menstrual fluid.

The disposable forms are to be placed in trash receptacles as these items can cause major plumbing issues when flushed. At the time of this writing the authors consulted a licensed Master Plumber with over 25 years in the industry covering Central and Southeastern Pennsylvania. He shared the following costs to unclog a toilet from flushing a hygiene product, during typical daytime business hours. Just to unclog a toilet blocked by a hygiene product is between $100 - $200. If the product got caught in the plumbing system pump it would cost approximately $750 to unjam and an additional $1,500 to $10,000 to replace the pump. Mainline blockages can cost between $350 to $700 to clear. If deficiencies are found in the mainline blockage sewer replacement costs range from $4,500 to over $60,000. Add these costs to having stalls closed for repair or even bathrooms closed because of blockages. If you were at a location and had to use the restroom only to find it was closed for plumbing repairs, what would you do, how would you feel?

MENSTRUAL CYCLE PHASES

My friend had that situation happen... she was at a music festival on a hot summer day and nature called after she had a few bottles of water. Although the venue was a nice size, they only had one restroom with several stalls. She arrived at the restroom only to find a long, agitated line and several "Out of Order" signs taped to stall doors. A festival staff member explained that tampons were flushed down several toilets, causing a major blockage in the system. Now, a majority of the toilets are unusable, and a repair team is on the way—but who knows how long that will take as this is a weekend and outside regular business hours for the plumbing company. As she waited in the seemingly endless line, she couldn't help but think about how tiny misplaced hygiene products have inconvenienced hundreds of people, and almost caused her to wet her pants.

It's a stark reminder that tampons, pads, and other menstrual products always go in the waste bin. These products are designed to absorb liquid and expand, which means they can easily clog pipes and cause plumbing nightmares. By disposing of them correctly,

MENSTRUAL CYCLE PHASES

you're protecting the plumbing and also showing consideration for everyone who might need the restroom after you.

It is also highly recommended that you read the instructions included with any product chosen on a regular basis. Please follow these instructions when it comes to the frequency of replacing a used product. Your body, usage frequency, and product choice will change throughout your life. Each product below has many options, experiment and find the one that works best for you.

Hygiene Pad/Pantyliner:

A pad/pantyliner is a flat piece of cotton or cotton blend material attached to a liquid blocking bottom to hold menstrual fluid. There are disposable types of pads and there are reusable types. Disposable types usually have an open weave top layer, cotton or cotton blend middle, with plastic along the bottom that sticks to underwear. Reusable types are made with soft fabric on top and bottom with absorbing material in between.

This product is placed on the inside of your underwear between the legs covering the vulva. They come in several thicknesses and lengths, some have "wings" that will wrap around the underwear to keep in place. The disposable type stays in place using a sticky adhesive on the underside. The reusable type may sit in your undergarments or may attach to material like Velcro or snaps below the undergarment.

The pad absorbs the menstrual fluid as it exits the vaginal canal. Depending on menstrual flow this product can be worn between 30 minutes on very heavy days to 6 hours on very light days. It is highly suggested to change this product every 4-6 hours if menstruation is extremely light or if it is worn when not menstruating. To change the pad, gently pull up on the pad and push down on your undergarment to release the product and place a new one in your underwear. Disposable ones can be placed in waste receptacles, reusable are to be rinsed, washed, and dried by manufacturers instructions.

Pads and pantyliners provide external protection and backup for other internal products like tampons or menstrual cups. For some, pads offer a sense of security and ease of use compared to internal options. Here's one perspective:

While many of my friends prefer tampons or menstrual cups, I've always felt most comfortable and confident using pads when I have my period. I appreciate not having to insert anything internally - the thought of accidentally leaving a tampon in too long honestly makes me a bit squeamish. Pads also require less preparation and feel easier to keep track of throughout the day.

Sure, they can seem a little bulkier than other options, but the brands I use feel surprisingly thin and discreet underneath my clothes. I've never had issues with noticeable leaks or odors. For me, the convenience and sense of security pads provide are worth it. Whether I'm at school, work, running errands, training, or just relaxing at home, I can go about my regular routine without stressing about period mishaps.

I've tried period underwear too but found myself still wanting the extra protection and absorption of a traditional pad, especially on heavier days. While everyone has different needs, pads remain my go-to period product. They allow me to stay fresh, comfortable, and confident in managing my menstrual flow each month.

Tampon:

A tampon is a cotton, cotton blend, or rayon roll that may or may not have a string attached or an applicator. Instead of being worn in underwear like a pad/pantyliner, it is inserted into the vaginal canal/vagina. It absorbs the menstrual fluid as it exits the cervix. This product is suggested to be changed at least every 8 hours to minimize the risk of toxic shock syndrome, a rare yet deadly infection. To change a tampon, wash your hands, then gently pull on the string or pull the tampon from the vaginal canal. The vaginal canal is small and tampons can be found easily when ready to remove. Used tampons are to be thrown in waste receptacles. Many use tampons when swimming while having their period. Although using a tampon is acceptable up to 8 hours, it is suggested to use another hygiene product for overnight.

Tampons allow you to go about daily activities with more freedom and discretion. Many people prefer them, especially for certain occasions or activities. Here's one perspective on using tampons: As I get ready for my day, I reach into my period supplies and grab a tampon. For me, it's an easy choice over pads. Tampons allow me to go about my usual routine without feeling weighed down or worried about leaks. At school, I can sit through classes without shifting uncomfortably. At soccer practice, I can run, jump, and play without that bulky feeling. And when I'm out with friends, I don't have to obsessively check or feel self-conscious.

Tampons are also more discreet - no one has to know I'm on my period unless I choose to mention it. From an environmental standpoint, they produce less waste too. While pads work for some people, tampons just make my period feel like less of an inconvenience.

Of course, everyone has their preferences, and there's no one-size-fits-all. But being able to use tampons gives me confidence and freedom during that time of the month. I can put one in and

MENSTRUAL CYCLE PHASES

almost forget about my period for a while as I tackle whatever the day brings.

Menstrual cups or discs:

Cups or discs are reusable products made from a silicone base. They are flexible and collect menstrual fluid versus absorb the fluid from the cervix like pads and tampons. The cups are worn like a tampon, inside the vaginal canal, but they cover the cervical opening capturing the fluid as it leaves the uterus. Because the cup is collecting fluid, a cup or disc can be worn for 10 to 12 hours as they hold more fluid significantly reducing the risk of toxic shock syndrome. When removing a cup or disc, be careful as it will contain fluid. Cups and discs are suggested to be washed before reinsertion into the vaginal canal. It may take several months of usage to get used to wearing a menstrual cup or disc.

While they take some practice to get used to inserting, removing, and cleaning properly, many people find cups and discs to be a more eco-friendly, cost-effective, and comfortable option for period care. Here's one person's perspective after using a menstrual cup for over a year:

While reusable menstrual cups and discs seemed daunting at first, I'm so glad I gave them a try. Trying to figure out the right one for me was simple when I heard about the free cup size quiz from Put A Cup In It at https://putacupinit.com/quiz/. The quiz asked me questions about my period, age, activity level, health history, and gave me several suggestions on cups that would work for my body. There is also a separate disc quiz. The quiz took the guesswork away.

Those first few cycles, getting the insertion and removal right was definitely a learning curve. There were some messy moments as I figured out the proper angle and technique. But after a month or two of practice, using the cup became second nature.

Now, I almost forget I'm on my period when I have the cup in. No bunchy pads, no risk of leaks, and no need to constantly check or change products throughout the day. The cup just collects everything with ease. I can sleep through the night, exercise, and go

MENSTRUAL CYCLE PHASES

about my normal routine without worries. Emptying it twice a day is so simple.

From an environmental perspective, I love producing virtually no waste each month. And financially, using the same medical-grade silicone cup cycle after cycle has saved me bundles compared to disposable product costs. While cups aren't for everyone, they've been a game-changer for my comfort and confidence during my period. I'll never go back to pads or tampons!

Period Underwear:

This is a relatively new period product. They look, feel, and wear like traditional underwear, however, have a very absorbent gusset (area that covers the vulva) versus regular underwear that is only a few layers of cloth. This product eliminates or reduces the use of other period products like pads, tampons, or cups.

A period underwear review: When I first tried period underwear, I was a bit skeptical about how secure and comfortable it would actually feel. It's so freeing not to worry about changing pads or tampons constantly. The moisture-wicking fabric keeps me feeling dry and fresh. No more ruining my clothes or sheets!

Aside from the convenience factor, I love how much waste I'm preventing by not using disposable products every month. Period underwear is better for the environment and costs less in the long run too. But most of all, it's given me peace of mind to manage my period without stressing over changing products in inconvenient situations. Period underwear has been a total game-changer!

A second perspective from a mom whose daughter just started getting her period. When my daughter got her first period, I wanted to make sure she felt prepared but not overwhelmed. We packed period underwear in her school bag just in case, and it has been a total game changer. Knowing she has a comfortable, reliable resource with her gives her so much confidence. No more worrying about leaks or rushing to the bathroom—she can focus on her day without stress. It's been such a relief for both of us during this new stage!

MENSTRUAL CYCLE PHASES

There's one additional thing to consider before we end this section. Accidents happen, bleeding can be heavier than expected and the product that we've used for years can fail. So be prepared, have a bag with you in your locker, car, or backpack that has an extra pair of stretch pants, underwear, hygiene products of several sizes, and cleansing or baby wipes to clean yourself. Trust me it will save you from having a traumatically embarrassing moment like this one...

I arrived at school in a nice sweater and dark dress pants. My period had started the night before, so it was a little on the heavier side, nothing out of the ordinary and I made sure I had plenty of pads with me for the day. I arrived at my first class after homeroom, every thing went wonderfully well until I went to stand up at the end of class and felt a gush; looked at my chair and saw a bright red blood spot. I knew instantly I sprung a leak! I quickly made my way to the restroom hoping my hygiene product was just full enough to leak a little bit. Nope, my pants were covered in blood, my underwear were unusable without major washing. I had a minute or two between

MENSTRUAL CYCLE PHASES

classes before I was late, plus I only wore pads at the time and there was no way I was standing in a bathroom with blood dripping down my leg washing and drying my underwear and pants. So, I did the next best thing. I cleaned up as best I could, placing toilet paper in my blood saturated underwear to absorb any new blood, and went immediately to the nurse's office. Now this was a time before cell phones were common or even available outside of cars. The only way to call home was from the school office or if there was a pay phone (it required the user to insert coins to make calls) in the school, most didn't have this or it was in a really inconvenient place. The nurse was a lovely, matured woman who listened to my story and began collecting several items so I could return to class. She grabbed a spare pair of disposable hospital underwear, a massive super absorbency pad that looked and felt like a pool noodle, and a pair of WHITE sweatpants. Everyone who saw me earlier that day knew something had happened. It was super embarrassing and over 30 years later is still traumatic. Yet a great learning tool to show how having a small kit with you can be empowering.

MENSTRUAL CYCLE PHASES

FOLLICULAR

Thought For This Phase: *New beginnings are unfolding within me. I am nurturing my body and cultivating energy for growth. I move with grace and vitality, aligning my actions with my desires and dreams.*

As menstruation ends, FSH decreases to pre-menstruation levels and estrogen begins rising as we enter the follicular growth section. This rise in estrogen is causing several ovarian follicles to grow and your uterine lining to grow as well. Several follicles begin a race to maturity with the winner being the largest and ovulated from the follicle into the fallopian tube. The remaining follicles die and are reabsorbed by the ovary.

During this phase you may notice your energy levels are really starting to rise, and you are able to do more in less time. You may notice trouble sleeping or that you are becoming super focused on school or an activity during this time. You can do more things now than you could a few days or even a week ago. You may be more social and want to spend time more time with friends and meet

MENSTRUAL CYCLE PHASES

new people. This is a great time to do these types of activities. As an athlete or high achiever this is the perfect time to focus on skill development, new trainings and the little things that create the biggest impacts in your performance. Some things you may notice about your body in this phase, your energy is higher, your clothing begins to feel looser, your skin might be clearer or have less acne or blemishes. Foods to help support your body during this phase include dark leafy greens, black eyed peas, carrots, zucchini, avocado, citrus fruits, cashews, chicken, and liver.

The follicular section of your cycle can last 4 to 7 days in a 28 day cycle, or it can be over 20 days in a 36 day cycle. The length of this section and the phase depends on many factors like stress, illness, medications, excessive exercise, and poor nutrition, just to name a few major ones.

You'll know if this phase will be a longer one when the cervical mucus changes later in this section. At the beginning of the follicular section, when wiping it might feel dry after menstruation. The dryness will begin changing to feeling more moisture or

4 Types of Cervical Mucus

Dry

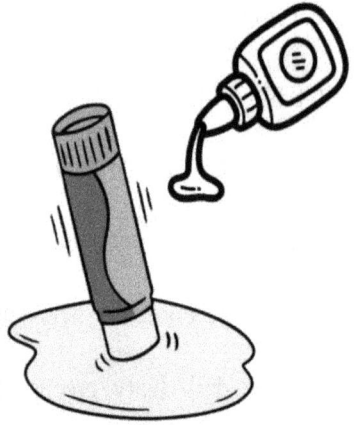

Paste/Sticky

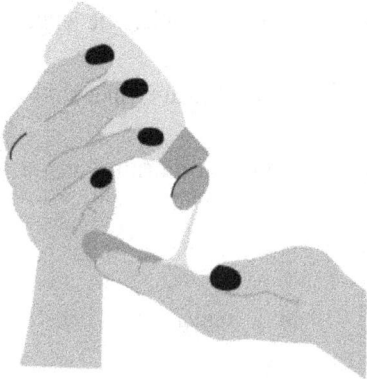

Lotion

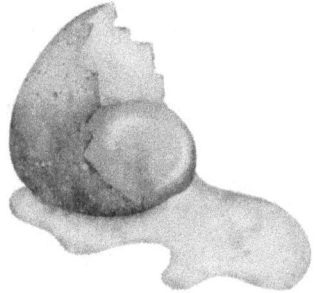

Clear/Stretchy/ Slippery

MENSTRUAL CYCLE PHASES

wetness when wiping during the middle days of this section. This is typical and healthy, what you are seeing is cervical mucus. Cervical mucus is a fluid produced by the cervix in reaction to hormonal changes throughout the menstrual cycle. It is an important biomarker and observation that indicates healthy hormonal health. Cervical mucus comes in several colors, mostly white, light grey, light yellow or transparent. The closer one gets to ovulation, the more moisture and wetness one feels when wiping. As ovulation approaches the more transparent, slippery, and stretchy the cervical mucus will become. Any cervical mucus that is a dark yellow, green, or other color could be an indication of an infection, especially if itching and burning sensations are noticed. If this is experienced, please seek guidance from your coach, parent, and a medical professional.

This section ends when your cervical mucus production goes from dry to feeling wet like a lotion to a clear, slippery, stretchy mucus that looks like raw egg whites. When your cervical mucus changes to the clear, stretchy, slippery cervical mucus, estrogen has hit a high point in your cycle and ovulation will possibly occur in the next two to three days. This time frame from feeling dry to feeling and seeing cervical mucus is when you've reached the transition into your ovulation section, the last portion of the follicular phase. This is also the time in your cycle when you are the most fertile.

OVULATION

Thought For This Phase: *I am a wellspring of vitality and enthusiasm. My energy levels are soaring, propelling me toward my biggest dreams. I move through life with confidence and radiant joy. This is a time to celebrate my strength and soak up every moment of exhilaration. I am grateful for the power flowing through me.*

This is the final section of the first half of your cycle. There have been significant changes in your hormonal levels and the ovarian follicles since the first day of menstruation. The follicles that began growing earlier in the follicular section are now competing for which ovum (egg) will be the biggest and get the chance to be released from the follicle into the fallopian tube at ovulation. The ovulation section in the follicular phase is the main event of your cycle, it lasts about 3-4 days. This is when estrogen hits its highest point during your cycle, the pituitary gland releases LH, that LH release causes the most mature ovarian follicle to open up and spit out an egg. You may experience some spotting or cramping during this time. This can be a typical response of ovulation for you, as hormones can fluctuate 30-50% over these few days. If you have pain-free ovulation, that is healthy too.

The ovulated egg will only live for about 12-24 hours, unless it is fertilized. The other maturing follicles in the ovary for that month will shrink and be absorbed by your body. Many sources state ovulation occurs around cycle day 14, in an average 28 day cycle. This might be true for some, for others ovulation occurs on or around different days. So, if you have an average 28 day cycle, ovulation may occur between cycle day 10 and cycle day 19. This is where tracking and being observant of your unique cycle comes in handy.

During this final section you are looking and feeling even more unstoppable, your skin is glowing, clothes fit better, you are feeling on top of the world. Go out and enjoy life. This is a great time to do a presentation, ask for a promotion, give a big sales pitch, perform on stage, or hit a high personal record. A word of caution, this is a high-risk time for injuries though, so be careful. Foods to help support your body during this phase include brussel sprouts, asparagus, raspberries, red lentils, shrimp, beef, dandelion, tomato, and pistachios.

After ovulation occurs, the follicle that released the mature egg develops into a new temporary organ called the corpus luteum. This corpus luteum has a crucial role: to produce progesterone, often referred to as the "calming, feel-good hormone."

LUTEAL

Thought For This Phase: *I am in harmony with the changing tides within. I give myself permission to pause, reflect, and replenish. I treat my body and emotions with tenderness, allowing space to integrate these natural shifts.*

Once ovulation occurs your body has moved into the final half of your cycle and last phase, called the Luteal phase. LH has returned to pre-ovulation levels, estrogen has decreased a little bit from ovulation levels, yet remains high, and progesterone is rising until approximately seven days after ovulation.

Progesterone is vital for maintaining bone and brain health, relaxing blood vessels, normalizing breast tissue, promoting sleep and relaxation, decreasing anxiety, and stabilizing the uterine lining until menstruation begins.

As you enter the luteal phase, your body starts to wind down from the super-charged energy of ovulation. Think of it like shifting from a big final performance to a post-performance wrap up meeting or practice. This is your body's way of saying, "Let's take it easy!" You might feel like doing slower activities - maybe some light yoga, a walk, or swimming. It's okay to spend more time relaxing, watching movies with friends or family, or just hanging out.

Your emotions and thoughts might feel a bit like a roller coaster too. You might suddenly want to spend money on something big or feel unsure about yourself - and that's completely normal! Sometimes your brain and hormones play these little tricks on you.

MENSTRUAL CYCLE PHASES

The cool part is, now you know what's happening, so you can be kind to yourself and give you and your teammates grace.

Your body might start sending some interesting signals during this time. You could feel extra hungry and find yourself craving specific foods like something sweet, salty, or with a strong taste. Sometimes you might feel a bit more tired than usual, and you could be more likely to catch a cold. What many people call "PMS" is actually your body's way of telling you that something might be out of balance with your hormones. Your body might feel different too - maybe your clothes feel a bit tighter, or you might see some acne showing up. These symptoms - like bloating, headaches, or mood swings - are like little warning lights on a car dashboard, signaling that your hormonal system might need some extra attention and care. These aren't just random changes, but potential signs that your hormones aren't working together as smoothly as they could. Understanding these signals is super important because they can give you early insights into your overall hormonal health. By paying attention now, you can learn how to support your body and potentially prevent more serious menstrual issues down the road.

To help your body feel its best, try eating foods that can make you feel good. Bananas are awesome for giving you energy, chickpeas can help you feel full, and dark chocolate can boost your mood, but also give you a needed nutrient called magnesium. Other great foods include squash, fish, turkey, and walnuts. Think of these as your body's superhero fuel!

The most important thing to remember? All of these feelings and changes are part of your amazing body's natural cycle, and they'll pass in a few days.

Inside your body the egg that was ovulated is traveling through the fallopian tubes the first

Only around 3% of the worlds biological female population knows how to track their cycle to know their unique pattern. We highly encourage you to be one of them!

four to five days of this phase before arriving in the uterus. During its travels, hormones are communicating between the egg and corpus luteum telling the corpus luteum to continue producing progesterone. If the egg was fertilized it will attempt to attach itself

MENSTRUAL CYCLE PHASES

to the plush endometrial lining and continue to communicate with the corpus luteum for another 10 to 12 weeks until a new organ called the placenta is made. If fertilization fails to occur at ovulation (which is what happens during a majority of cycles), the egg will stop communicating with the corpus luteum after seven or eight days. The stopping of communication tells the corpus luteum to discontinue making progesterone. When the corpus luteum stops making progesterone, levels will begin dropping and menstruation will begin in approximately five to seven days.

The beautiful thing about these phases and the body is that all of this that we just covered can be tracked in about one to two minutes each day. It is so simple, plus it gives you a chance to see cycle patterns. The patterns will become clearer as time passes and any changes to the pattern will show up so medical attention can be scheduled with possible diagnostics, decreasing the potential severity and length of the condition. Only around 3% of the worlds biological female population knows how to track their cycle to know their unique pattern. We highly encourage you to be one of them!

MENSTRUAL CYCLE PHASES

Summary:

- The menstrual cycles is made up of two halves containing four phases, menstruation, follicular, ovulation, and luteal
- Biomarkers are important indicators of health
- Hygiene products come in all shapes, sizes, and options both internal and external

MENSTRUAL CYCLE PHASES

CYCLICAL LIVING : A MONTH IN FLOW

LUTEAL PHASE: WHAT?

Autumn = Waning Moon
High Progestrone & Estrogen

Energy Decreases   Finish up projects
May experience imposter
syndrome & trouble focusing

Snuggling and connecting

Dark chocolate, high fiber, &
high protein

OVULATORY PHASE: DO!
Summer = Full Moon
High Estrogen & Testosterone
High Confidence Go Have FUN!
Step out of comfort zone
High Energy & pain tolerance
Shrimp, beef, tomato, asparagus

*Follicle Stimulating Hormone

MENSTRUAL PHASE: WHY?

Winter = New Moon
Low Progesterone and Estrogen, Rising FSH*

Low Energy   Self care
minimal thinking tasks, filing,
cleaning out email
Manifesting   Gentle stretching
Reading and journal
Soups, cranberries, ham, ginger
tea, dark leafy vegetables

FOLLICULAR PHASE: HOW?
Spring = Waxing Moon
Rising Estrogen & Lutenizing Hormone
Increasing Energy   Learn, Grow, Plan
Insomnia   High Productivity
HIIT, Increase exercise intensity
Lemons, broccoli, zucchini, carrots

MENSTRUAL CYCLE PHASES

CYCLE TRACKING FOR CLARITY
AND CONFIDENCE

I'm sure you've heard of people suggesting tracking cycles. There are so many ways to do this. The most basic way is marking a calendar on the first day of red bleeding and then marking the calendar again when the next cycle restarts. This is a good very basic beginning method; however, this method leaves a lot of vital information out. As we learned earlier hormones fluctuate, and when they do, they give outward signals called biomarkers. Biomarkers provide a clearer picture of what is happening with hormones inside the body. These biomarkers change as one moves through the monthly cycle. Some examples of biomarkers include menstruation, cervical mucus, basal body temperature, cervical position, and cervical texture. Other vital biomarkers our body provides are heart rate, blood pressure, and temperature.

We can track cycle biomarkers on paper or on apps. Apps have been a popular option for many years. They are easy, convenient, and usually always on hand. The few drawbacks, to be aware of, with apps are their use of algorithms and the potential of a third party getting ahold of your personal health information.

Apps are designed to calculate arrival of periods and ovulation using an average 28-day cycle with ovulation being around day 14. If your cycle is outside the average 28-day cycle or it has a different time frame for ovulation, it could take years of data to recalculate and give a better understanding of your cycle because of the algorithms. Some apps also miss the opportunity to enter biomarker observations, which can begin to show important cycle data outside just bleeding and cervical mucus.

Paper on the other hand is a less than ideal option as it can be a little more cumbersome. We must remember to grab our tracker or place it somewhere it will be handy to remind us to enter the data on a regular basis. It takes a little more planning, yet can give significantly more accurate data. This is why I prefer the paper over apps, however see which works best for you. There is an app I like to use that does provide space for data like the paper, it is free and through a science based organization at FEMMhealth.org.

No matter how tracking is done, we encourage turning tracking into a daily habit by doing it at the same time every day, like part of a bedtime routine. In addition to becoming a habit, this tracking method is different than almost every other tracker on the market. The method explained in this section is an education-based method from a reproductive health plan, meaning it was researched and designed by experts in biological female reproductive health and taught to others who specialize in biological female health. It can help provide medical professionals with more accurate information and better knowledge of how to best incorporate treatment if you develop menstrual disorder(s). Statistics show 9 out of 10 biological females have at least one or more menstrual issues during their lifetime. I've included examples using the paper tracker, however the app works in a very similar way, except it is missing the moon, emotion, competition, and monthly intention sections.

On the enclosed Period Tracker pages, cycle days are along the top, then date, next line down is moon phase, flow color, your daily emotion, a space to mark if you competed that day, and a notes section. Your charting can begin on any day of your cycle with Chart 1. We encourage you to start tracking as soon as possible. This gets you into a habit and also begins your in-depth knowledge of your body. You could start recognizing patterns as soon as the first full cycle, or it may take two or three cycles to really see a pattern develop, depending on how your cycle works. If you would like help with paper tracking or learning how to track that assists you in becoming an informed medical advocate for

> Statistics show 9 out of 10 biological females have at least one or more menstrual issues during their lifetime.

yourself and hitting your goals; check out the XXStrong membership. We offer in-depth guidance on tracking, mindset, nutrition, and more. Helping you understand how hormonal changes affect your performance and provide the tools you need to excel, empowering yourself with knowledge to elevate your game.

HOW TO USE THIS CHART:

During the day, keep note of how it feels when you wipe from front to back after using the restroom. Wiping front to back is good hygiene practice, it also allows you to better feel the cervical mucus across the perineum. The perineum is a small area of skin with many nerve endings between the vaginal opening and the rectum. It is very sensitive to feeling moisture. At the end of the day, write down the date, the current moon phase in the sky, the biomarker color of the highest estrogenic mucus you experienced throughout the day, even if it was only once, your overall emotion for the day, if you had a competition that day, and notes like medication changes or new/stopped medication, high stress days, heavy training days, illness, PMS symptoms, number of product changes that day, flow volume when menstruating, etc. All of this is important and will help you see patterns as you track. Again, if you need more help learning how to track check out the XXStrong membership, information can be found in the resources section of the book.

Biomarker colors:

This tracker requires writing down biomarkers of menstruation and cervical mucus. There are colors and symbols listed below that will help make this process easy and convenient. As stated earlier, this process is a one to two minute per day process. A video on how to begin charting and a full month of charting can be found here:

CYCLICAL LIVING : A MONTH IN FLOW

LUTEAL PHASE: WHAT?

Autumn = Waning Moon
High Progestrone & Estrogen

Energy Decreases Finish up projects
May experience imposter
syndrome & trouble focusing

Snuggling and connecting

Dark chocolate, high fiber, &
high protein

OVULATORY PHASE: DO!

Summer = Full Moon
High Estrogen & Testosterone
High Confidence Go Have FUN!
Step out of comfort zone
High Energy & pain tolerance
Shrimp, beef, tomato, asparagus

*Follicle Stimulating Hormone

MENSTRUAL PHASE: WHY?

Winter = New Moon
Low Progesterone and Estrogen, Rising FSH*

Low Energy   Self care
minimal thinking tasks, filing,
cleaning out email
Manifesting   Gentle stretching

Reading and journal
Soups, cranberries, ham, ginger
tea, dark leafy vegetables

FOLLICULAR PHASE: HOW?

Spring = Waxing Moon
Rising Estrogen & Lutenizing Hormone
Increasing Energy Learn, Grow, Plan
Insomnia   High Productivity
HIIT, Increase exercise intensity
Lemons, broccoli, zucchini, carrots

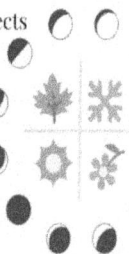

During menstruation the following colors and symbols will help bring the tracker to life. Some may find some additional colors are needed during menstruation. This does happen. When it does split the flow space for the day in half, so half is red and the other half of the square is the other color. The video showing tracking will have an example.

Red: this is the color used for all menstruation. In the notes section indicate how many product changes were done that day and volume of flow using the following list:

- H: Heavy (5+ changes that day)

- M: Medium (3-4 product changes that day)

- L: Light (2-3 product changes that day)

- S: spotting (1 or less product changes that day)

- B: Brown

After menstruation is complete, the colors below are to indicate cervical mucus for the remainder of the month. These colors may also be used during menstruation, if noticed. A sample of this is in the how to track YouTube video here:

Day	1	2	3	4	5	6	7	8	9	10	11	12	13	14	15	16	17	18	19	20	21	22	23	24	25	26	27	28	29	30	31	32	33	34	35	36	37	38	39	40
Date																																								
Moon																																								
Flow	H	H	M	L																																				
Emotion																																								
Compete	Y		Y																																					
Notes	5	5	3	2																																				

Monthly Intentions

The first few days of your period is the perfect time to set intentions for the month. It is suportive of new beginnings and fresh starts. Write down your hopes, dreams, and goals using "I will or I am" statements

CYCLE TRACKING FOR CLARITY AND CONFIDENCE

Light Blue: This color is used when cervical mucus feels like lotion or wetness when wiping.

Dark Blue: This color is used when cervical mucus is clear, slippery, and stretchy.

Grey: This color is used when there is dryness when wiping.

Yellow: This color is used when cervical mucus feels tacky, sticky, or an odd color. This color may also be mixed with blue or red, depending on your cycle and hormones. When using this color, write in the notes section if there is any unusual smell, itching or burning either while urinating or when not using the restroom.

To begin tracking we've tried to keep it super simple. Go to Chart 1, write the date in the date section, look at a calendar and write in the moon phase (new, waxing, full, or waning), at the end of the day fill in the flow space with the correct color (red, grey, shade of blue, yellow, or a mixture of these). Any days you feel dry when wiping, mark grey, any feelings of moisture or wetness use light blue, slippery/gooey mark in dark blue, any unsure days mark yellow, menstruation days are red with the correct symbol in the notes section, and choose your own emotion color (from the included Emotion Wheel). Track this way until your period begins and then mark your first continuous red bleeding day under day 1 in red on the next chart. Continue tracking as above.

If you get to day 40 on the chart and you still haven't started a period yet, go to the next chart under day 1. Once your period arrives, start a new chart on day 1. Count how many days past day 45 and mark it at the end margin of your chart so you know how long your cycles are lasting.

When starting a new chart, count how many days you colored grey from dark blue. This will give you an idea on how long your luteal phase is. An example of charting can be found on our YouTube channel at https://youtu.be/rxILJVBYGn4 or by scanning this QR code:

The Moon/Period Connection:

Interestingly, there is evidence to suggest that moon phases may influence menstrual cycles in some individuals. Some studies have found correlations between moon cycles and the timing of ovulation and menstruation, although the mechanisms behind this phenomenon are not yet fully understood. While not all women experience a moon influence on their cycles, it's a fascinating aspect to consider and may provide additional insight into the mysterious rhythms of the female body.

For those who are currently not menstruating or have reached menopause, moon charting is a great way to see how your energy still ebbs and flows, much like how those that are still menstruating. For those that are menstruating, including the moon will allow you to visually connect the moon to where you are in your cycle. Some individuals may notice menstruation is at new moon, where others may menstruate during other moon phases. Where your menstruation and the moon line up is unique and perfect for you. As time goes on this lining of the moon and menstruation will probably change, however it is a really interesting pattern to be aware of because each moon phase correlates to the cycle phases from the earlier chapter.

MENSTRUAL PHASE: WHY?

Winter = New Moon

Low Progesterone and Estrogen

Low Energy

Self care

Filing, cleaning out email, minimal thinking tasks

Manifesting

Gentle stretching

Reading and journal

Soups, cranberries, ham, ginger tea, dark leafy vegetables

FOLLICULAR PHASE: HOW?

Spring = Waxing Moon

Rising *FSH, Estrogen, & LH

Increasing Energy

Learn, Grow, Plan

Insomnia

High Productivity

HIIT, Increase exercise intensity

Lemons, broccoli, zucchini, carrots

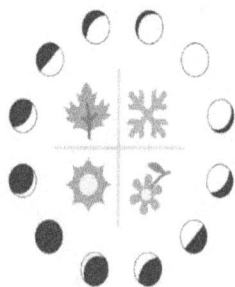

As we learned earlier, our cycle has phases and so does the moon. Each moon phase corresponds to different activities. Almost all phases of the moon have journal prompts, except the full moon, that is a DO phase versus journalling.

The New Moon is associated with menstruation, intentions, and the beginnings of a new cycle. This is a great time to set intentions for the month ahead. The new moon encourages new beginnings and fresh starts. Meditation and journalling are great activities to engage in during this time. Some essential oils that may help with emotions and symptoms during this time include ylang ylang, clary sage, grapefruit and herbal scents like oregano and thyme. Your body may want to hear simple calming music.

The Waxing /First Quarter Moon is paired with the follicular section of the cycle. It is a great time to conceptualize, focus on detail, begin new projects, learn new things, refine current projects, and being patient. Some essential oils that may help during this phase include citrus oils, oregano, juniper, and clove. Your body is starting to like action movies and music that induces movement and dancing.

OVULATORY PHASE: DO!

Summer = Full Moon

High Estrogen & Testosterone

High Confidence

Go Have FUN!

Step out of comfort zone

High Energy & pain tolerance

Shrimp, beef, tomato, asparagus

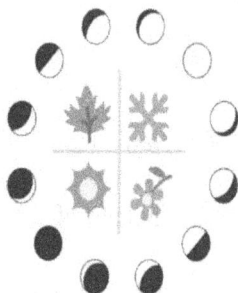

LUTEAL PHASE: WHAT?

Autumn = Waning Moon

High Progestrone & Estrogen

Energy Decreases

Finish up projects

May experience imposter
syndrome & trouble focusing

Snuggling and connecting

Dark chocolate, high fiber, &
high protein

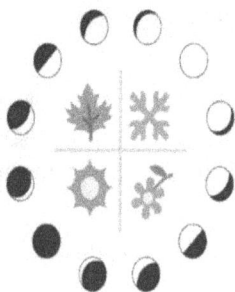

The Full Moon is partnered with ovulation. It reveals where you are with your intentions set at New Moon, allows you to receive the reveal, and it is also a great time for joy, gratitude, celebration, and you are at your peak energy. Some essential oils to use during this time include grapefruit, cypress, cinnamon, and geranium. Your body wants to move, go out and have fun with family and friends.

The Waning Moon is a time to harvest what you started earlier in your cycle, it is a time to transition, forgive, reflect, surrender, and nurture. Some essential oils to use during this time include ylang ylang, lavender, clary sage, and roman chamomile. Your body may want to do activities however you may get tired easily. It's a great time to snuggle on the couch with loved ones.

How does your cycle match up to the moon? Do your feelings and activities match or are you in alignment with a different moon phase? Once the moon phase is recorded, its onto the emotions. Emotions can vary throughout the day. In the next section look at which emotion stayed the longest throughout the day. You're welcome to split the box with several colors, this chart is uniquely yours.

In the emotions section:

First take some time to color the emotion wheel on page **139**.

Once the wheel is colored, look at the emotion wheel, find your emotion, and color the block in the period tracker on that day the same color as your emotion(s). Again, this block may have several colors depending on how you are feeling that day, use up to two strongly felt emotions throughout the day.

We include the emotion wheel because it is a powerful tool designed to help individuals identify and understand their emotions more effectively. At its core, the emotion wheel consists of a circular diagram divided into sections, each representing a different emotion or feeling. These emotions are often categorized into primary and secondary emotions, providing a comprehensive range of feelings that individuals may experience.

For athletes the emotion wheel can be particularly beneficial in helping navigate the complex emotional landscape that comes with competitive sports. Athletes may encounter a wide range of feelings, from excitement and confidence to frustration and anxiety, both on and off the field.

Using the emotion wheel, you can learn to recognize and label your emotions more accurately,

which is the first step in developing emotional intelligence. By pinpointing specific emotions, you can gain insight into the underlying reasons behind their feelings and begin to develop strategies for managing them effectively.

To use the emotion wheel effectively, follow these simple steps:

Identify the Emotion:

Take a moment to pause and reflect on how you're feeling in a given situation. Use the emotion wheel as a guide to identify the primary emotion that best describes your current state.

Explore Secondary Emotions:

Once you've identified the primary emotion, explore the surrounding sections of the emotion wheel to see if any secondary emotions resonate with you. Secondary emotions often provide additional context and depth to your initial feelings.

The Emotion Wheel

To color in the wheel, start with the pieces in the middle. Pick a color for each triangular center wedge, "Sad, Mad, Scared, Joyful, Powerful, Peaceful". Each of these colors will be the brightest color on the wheel. Once a color is decided for each of those, choose a slightly less bright shade of the same color for the six emotions attached to the center triangular color. Once this is complete, decide on a very light shade of each chosen color for the final 12 spaces connected to the center triangular piece.

Example: Joyful is bright yellow, the second segment of 6 spaces that includes "Excited" is a sunshine yellow, the third section of 12 spaces including "Amused" is a pale yellow.

To view a coloring demo of the Emotion Wheel, please visit XX Strong's YouTube Channel or scan the QR Code that will take you directly there.

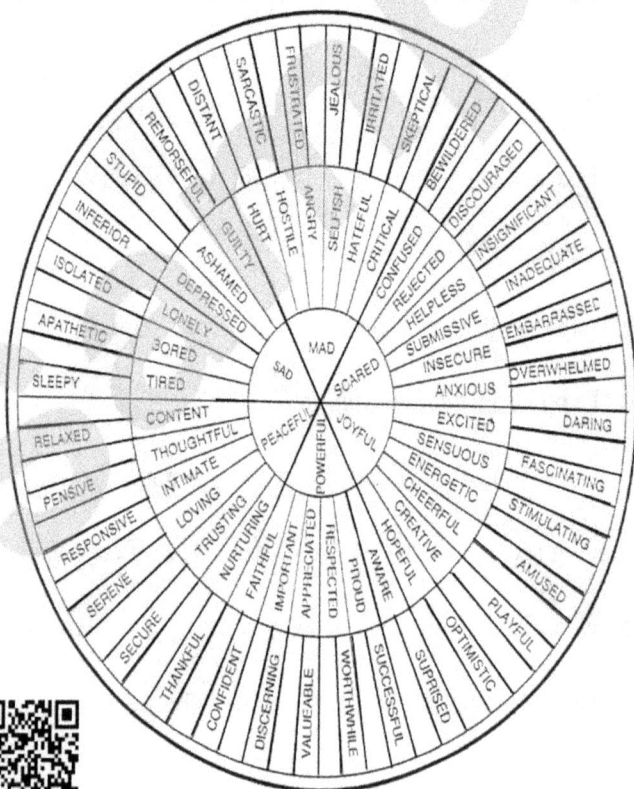

Developed by Dr. Gloria Wilcox

Validate and Reflect:

Acknowledge and validate your emotions without judgment. Remember that all emotions are valid and serve a purpose. Reflect on why you might be feeling a certain way and consider how your emotions are impacting your thoughts, behaviors, and performance.

Develop Coping Strategies:

Once you've identified your emotions, brainstorm healthy coping strategies to manage them effectively. This could include techniques such as deep breathing, visualization, positive self-talk, or seeking support from coaches, teammates, F.I.X. Code Coach, or mental health professionals.

By incorporating the emotion wheel into your daily routines, we develop greater self-awareness, emotional regulation skills, and resilience, ultimately enhancing overall performance and well-being.

Tracking menstrual cycles is not only essential for understanding reproductive health but also for empowering us to take control of our bodies and overall well-being. By familiarizing yourself with the four main phases of the menstrual cycle, adopting tracking methods that work for you, and exploring the potential moon connection, you can gain a deeper understanding of your body's natural rhythms and optimize your health for a happier, healthier life. If the thought of the phase mentioned before each phase earlier in the book failed to resonate with you, please find ones that resonate and use them. As life changes, the current thought phrase may change and that is ok, find new ones that feel good in the moment. You may find several for each phase, I like to keep extra's on sticky notes and place them around my home.

As you continue using the tracker, patterns begin to appear. These patterns are very important to notice and pay attention to because a pattern change can indicate potential health issues in the reproductive system or in one or more of the other body systems we briefly discussed earlier. It's been mentioned several times throughout this book that periods are outward signs of inner health and that how periods present themselves can potentially indicate health conditions.

One of those conditions is energy deficiency. Energy deficiency is when an individual uses more energy than is eaten.

Humans get energy from the foods we eat, when we use more energy than we eat, we intentionally or unintentionally place our bodies into a position that can be dangerous, if left unchecked. Energy deficiency can be experienced by athletes and non-athletes alike. Some initial symptoms of energy deficiency include tiredness, lowered heart rate, dizziness upon standing, weight loss, and irregular or missing periods. Some of these symptoms feel great and give us the feeling of being healthy or at the top of our athletic game, that we are in peak condition. When in reality, energy deficiency is leading to damaging your body.

Summary:

- What to look for when tracking your cycle
- The Moon/Period Connection and usage
- How emotions play a role in tracking your cycle

Our menstrual cycles are our fifth vital sign - they are monthly OB/GYN visits without the weight checks, papergowns, and cold medical instruments.

--- *Heather Allmendinger*

RELATIVE ENERGY DEFICIENCY IN SPORTS

For many biological females, missed periods are often seen as a blessing, yet this could be the first warning of a larger issue called Relative Energy Deficiency in Sport (RED-S). According to Science Direct.com, "(RED-S) refers to a condition in which energy imbalance leads to impaired physiological function of multiple organ systems and expands on the diagnosis previously known as the Female Athlete Triad, a medical condition often observed in physically active girls and women. It involves any one or more of the following three components that are often interrelated: low energy availability (with or without disordered eating/eating disorder), menstrual dysfunction, and low bone mineral density."

This condition is rooted in several factors, including consuming too few calories for the amount of energy spent (restrictive eating patterns associated with fad diets or extreme weight loss measures), extremely high volume or high intensity training without adequate rest and recovery increasing energy demands, body image or societal pressures to maintain a certain body weight or appearance influencing eating behaviors, certain medical conditions such as gastrointestinal disorders or hormonal

What's Impacted with Relative Energy Deficiency in Sports

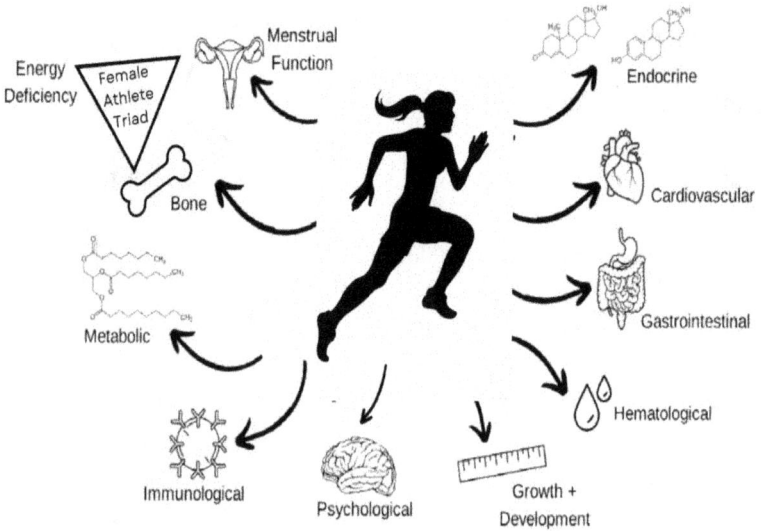

Energy Deficiency

Female Athlete Triad

Menstrual Function

Bone

Metabolic

Immunological

Psychological

Growth + Development

Hematological

Gastrointestinal

Cardiovascular

Endocrine

imbalances can interfere with energy metabolism, or a fixation around food (afraid to eat around others, fear of gaining weight if certain foods are eaten, using exercise to combat poor eating decisions). If left untreated it can be deadly or develop into lifelong health issues that can impact metabolic rate, hormones, immunity, and cardiovascular health. RED-S begins as fatigue, weight loss, missed periods, high rate of injury

RED-S can strike any highly active biological female whose energy intake falls short of her energy expenditure over time.

(stress fractures), reduced concentration, lack of response to training, reduced strength, and decreased endurance. One of the most severe forms of RED-S is missing 3 consecutive or more periods or starting a period at age 15 or older. While occasional cycle irregularity can occur due to stress, consistently missed periods after establishing a regular menstrual cycle is a critical red flag that warrants medical evaluation.

The statistics are sobering - estimates suggest RED-S affects a staggering 20% to 62% of female athletes across various sports and competitive levels. Among specific groups, the numbers are even higher - up to 44% of ballet dancers, 51% of endurance runners, and 44.8% of gymnasts may experience menstrual dysfunction.

Just ask Bernadine Bezuidenhout. At just 26 years old, the New Zealand wicketkeeper-batter was told her professional athletic career was over. Years without a period left her vomiting constantly, extremely weak, struggling to eat and sleep, with severe swelling. Her mindset of "the thinner, the better" had backfired drastically, causing her to develop full-blown RED-S by eating only 1,000 calories while burning 5,000 calories each day.

RED-S can strike any highly active biological female whose energy intake falls short of her energy expenditure over time. If you'll allow a quick personal story... In my high school years and into my early 20s, I was an active non-traditional athlete. I ate when hungry and thought I was perfectly healthy. Yet I experienced dizziness upon standing, severe menstrual cramps, coldness in extremities, and extremely low blood pressure readings that only slightly concerned doctors. Looking back, I likely had undiagnosed relative energy deficiency negatively impacting my overall health, I just didn't know it.

Our menstrual cycles are intimately connected to our overall health. It is a vital sign, it provides insights into complex biological processes. When energy intake plummets below the demands of training, it can disrupt this delicate balance, setting off a cascade of effects.

The risks of ignoring RED-S are substantial - decreased bone density, metabolic disturbances, weakened immunity, and long-term impacts on reproductive, cardiovascular, and mental health. One study found 100% of college cheerleaders showed symptoms of RED-S.

No athlete wants increased injury risk, lack of response to training, or a premature career end, and we don't have to accept these outcomes. By prioritizing education and open conversations, we can rewrite the narrative. Imagine embracing menstrual cycles as empowering

One of the most severe forms of RED-S is missing 3 consecutive or more periods or starting a period at age 15 or older. While irregular cycles can occur due to stress, consecutive missed periods after menstruation has started is a red flag.

insights to optimize performance, instead of obstacles. Where athletes confidently track cycles alongside biometrics, and coaches design individualized programs guided by an athlete's rhythms.

This journey starts with honest dialogues between athletes, parents, and professionals. Shifting our mindsets from viewing periods as inconvenient to treating them as vital signs of internal balance. Examining ingrained beliefs about thinness and societal pressures.

For those with RED-S symptoms, recovery is possible with guidance and support. Just look at Bezuidenhout, whose comeback after a decade without periods showcased the body's resilience. "I literally celebrated it...it was a massive achievement," she shared about her first period in years.

The path won't be easy, it will take a big shift in mindset, but the potential rewards are immense - optimized performance, reduced injuries, long-term positive health, and a newfound appreciation for being a biological female.

When experiencing menstrual issues such as missed or irregular periods, heavy painful cycles, long cycles, etc., it is common to visit medical professionals and be given the option of hormonal birth control to "fix" the possible issue. Medication is an easier route for some than looking at and changing the lifestyle. For those that choose medication over lifestyle changes, your own research is important to your current and future health. There are many options available, be informed of your risks, the pros and cons of the medication, long-term effects of the medication, and what is needed to stop or change if that particular medication falls outside your expectations or desires. Be sure to also ask your medical professional these questions. If left unsatisfied with the answers seek additional medical professional guidance. You are the biggest advocate of your own health.

The final chapter in this book is about the many different options of birth control and the nutrition suggestions to help support the body when dealing with negative menstrual symptoms like PMS, RED-S, and transitioning off of hormonal birth control. We have the right to be informed participants and advocates in our healthcare with the ability to make informed decisions. Informed choice is possible when learning and considering all the options and information available to make those empowered choices about our health after understanding how our bodies work. Now that you have some understanding of menstrual cycles, hormones, and how your body uses hormones in your cycles, let's look at the options you may have available.

Summary:

- What is Relative Energy Deficiency in Sports (RED-S)
- How to identify early symptoms
- Statistics of those impacted with RED-S

EMPOWERING CHOICE:

EXPLORING CONTRACEPTIVE OPTIONS

Deciding how best to care for your health can be a challenging decision. You've decided to visit a medical professional about some menstrual issues you're tired of dealing with and you're presented with a buffet of options.

You were presented with at least five contraception options spanning hormonal and non-hormonal approaches: short-term methods, long-term solutions, permanent procedures,

> You are the biggest advocate of your own health.

barrier techniques, and fertility awareness/education strategies. Each has a purpose, pros and cons, and effective rates both typical (average person usage) and perfect (following the medication instructions exactly as written), discontinuation rate (approximate percentage of users who have stopped taking a particular medication for method related reasons within a 12 month time frame), and monthly failure rate (approximate percentage of users who get pregnant using a particular contraceptive, with either perfect or typical use). With only one option that prevents sexually transmitted illness (STI), and that's the condom. Now before your head starts spinning, let's break these down a little more and explain very generally how they work and the forms available.

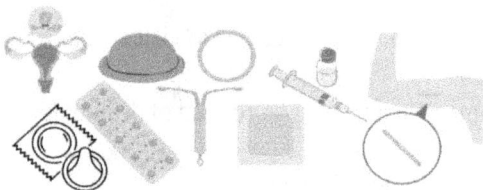

First let's start with hormonal versus non-hormonal. Hormonal birth control methods work by providing low levels of synthetic hormones to suppress natural hormonal activity in the body. They inhibit ovarian follicle development, attempt to prevent ovulation, thin the endometrial lining making it difficult for a fertilized egg to implant, and thicken cervical mucus, making it difficult for sperm to reach the uterus. These medications are the most widely prescribed medications for individuals with a uterus.

Non-hormonal birth control methods allow your body to produce and manage natural levels of hormonal activity in the body while attempting to prevent an ovulated egg reaching sperm. Ways this happen is through barriers, having a medical device inserted that is toxic to sperm, applying over the counter creams that kill sperm, or knowing your body's biomarkers to understand when you are ovulating and keeping sperm from entering the uterus. Menstrual cycles may change using some non-hormonal methods and those will be discussed a little later as each method is slightly different. Many of the non-hormonal methods can be purchased at the local store or online without medical professional approval.

Now that we know the difference between non-hormonal and hormonal birth control, let's look at the five different types, including pros/cons and prevention rate.

Short-Term Hormonal Contraception: Short-term hormonal contraception includes options such as the pill, , mini pill (progestin only), injectables, patches, and rings. They are hormonal in nature and require medical approval. These methods are effective for 3-4 weeks at a time and need replaced after that time. They require the user to use the medication consistently.

The Pill, Mini Pill, Ring, and Patch: The combined pill contains both a synthetic estrogen and progestin (a synthetic form of progesterone), while the mini pill is progestin-only. They are highly effective when taken each day at the same time. The typical 12-

EMPOWERING CHOICE: EXPLORING CONTRACEPTIVE OPTIONS

month failure rate is 9% for the pills, and the 12-month discontinuation rate of 33%. The typical 12 month failure rate is 9% for patches and ring, with a discontinuation rate of 44%.

Side effects can include menstrual irregularities, nausea, headaches, and mood changes. The low level of hormones can cause the menstrual cycle to halt while on this medication and thins out endometrial lining. During the 4th week of pills or removal of the ring or patch shedding of the endometrial lining may occur. This shedding happens because there is no medication being absorbed by the body to hold onto the lining. The bleeding is considered a breakthrough bleed or "fake" period.

Injectables: Injectable contraceptives like Depo-Provera are long-lasting forms of short-term contraception, with a typical failure rate of less than 1% and a 12 month discontinuation rate of 44%. The injection is performed by a medical practitioner every 12 weeks. Side effects of the medication include no periods, irregular menstrual bleeding, weight gain, headaches, abdominal pain/discomfort, mood disorders, bloating, acne, leg cramps, backaches, baldness, hot flashes, joint pain, convulsions, increased allergies or sensitivities, and disturbed liver function. Once this medication is stopped, it could take up to 24 months for a period to return and for natural hormones to return to healthy levels.

Long-Term Hormonal Contraceptives include the Intrauterine Devices (IUD). The IUD comes in hormonal and non-hormonal varieties. The hormonal IUDs, like Mirena, release low levels of levonorgestrel, a form of progestin, that prevents pregnancy and can stay in the body for up to 6-7 years. Copper IUDs are non-hormonal and work by being toxic to sperm, they can stay inside the body for up to 10 years. Both have a typical failure rate of less than 1% and a discontinuation rate of 16-22%. IUDs require a healthcare professional's insertion, and some side effects include menstrual changes, pelvic discomfort/pelvic inflammatory disease,

question your medical professional on side effects, effective rates, statistics, length of effectiveness, maximum length of using any type of birth control.

and rare complications such as the body pushing the IUD out or holes develop in the uterine or cervical wall.

Depending on the medication chosen and how the body reacts to the medication, an individual might experience heavy bleeding, breakthrough bleeding, spotting, or no period while taking any version of the above medications. Some general side effects and risks noted by almost all hormonal contraceptive methods include, depression, bone demineralization, infertility, blood clots, higher tendency to experience stroke and/or heart attack, increased chances of liver, breast, and cervical cancer.

The one condition that is very rarely mentioned or thought of when using any form of hormonal birth control is delayed cervical maturation. The cervix has a single layer of skin to protect it until puberty. Once puberty begins the cervix starts to grow additional layers of skin to protect itself and the uterus from infections. By the time a biological female hits the early 20's the cervix will grow up to 30 skin layers thick, however, the usage of hormonal birth control delays this protective growth increasing the risk of sexually transmitted diseases (STIs). The population with the highest diagnosis of STIs is 15-25 years of age.

Now there is a way to protect against most STIs in the non-hormonal group. We recently finished the hormonal methods available, below are the non-hormonal methods, except for the copper IUD that was covered in the hormonal section.

Non-Hormonal Barrier Methods: Barrier methods, such as condoms, diaphragms, and cervical caps, prevent sperm from reaching the uterus. These methods are non-hormonal but should be used in conjunction with spermicides for increased effectiveness. Condoms are single use and the only form of contraception that also protects against STI. They can be purchased at most stores. Diaphragms and cervical caps require a medical professional approval for purchasing. Failure rates of typical usage over the course of a year vary between methods, condoms having a failure rate of 2%, diaphragms have a 13% failure rate, and cervical caps have a 14% failure rate. It's important to note that some individuals may experience allergies, irritation, or increased risk of urinary tract infections using these types of methods.

Sterilization: Sterilization methods, such as tubal ligation, a surgical procedure involving cutting or blocking the fallopian tubes to prevent eggs from reaching sperm, offers semi-permanent birth control. While highly effective at preventing pregnancy, it is usually considered irreversible, however reversal is possible. If reversed, the successful conception rate is between 30-50%. Permanent sterilization for a biological female is through a partial hysterectomy (where the uterus and fallopian tubes are removed keeping at least one ovary intact) or full hysterectomy where the uterus, fallopian tubes, and both ovaries are removed. Full hysterectomies are now uncommon unless medically necessary.

Fertility awareness methods: These methods include tracking menstrual cycles and observing biomarkers such as cervical mucus, cervical position, basal body temperature,

> "Knowledge-based methods educate an individual to understand the science and signs of their body. All other methods leave one uninformed."
>
> -Fertility Education & Medical Management

and using ovulation prediction strips. It does require dedication and accuracy, but can be an effective hormone-free alternative. Some methods include calendar method, rhythm method, Sympto-Thermal, Creighton's, Billings, and FEMM. These methods are also a wonderful way to see what is happening within your bodily systems. A period is a visit to a medical practitioner every month minus the practitioner, scale, and gown. These methods have varying levels of effectiveness and require proper education and guidance. With proper education and guidance, they boast high levels of prevention within 3 months, the DIY (do it yourself) learner could take 6 months or longer to master the method. The FEMM method boasts a 93-98% effective rate, the same as the combination pill discussed under short-term hormonal methods. "Knowledge-based methods educate an individual to understand the science and signs of their body. All other methods leave one uninformed." - Fertility Education & Medical Management

Each of the methods listed above have pros/cons, effective rates, and require some sort of major decision on the part of the end user. Do your research and make the best decision for you and your body. It is very highly recommended to **question your medical professional on side effects, effective rates, statistics, length of effectiveness, maximum length of using any type of birth control.** If your medical provider gives answers that feel off to you, please request information from another provider. You must be the advocate for your own health.

By exploring the diverse range of contraception methods available, you have gained valuable insights into their pros, cons, and potential considerations. Remember that contraceptive choices should be made in consultation with healthcare professionals, considering factors such as effectiveness, side effects, and individual preferences. Whether you opt for hormonal options, non-hormonal methods, or fertility awareness-based approaches, informed choice and empowerment are key to making decisions that align with your reproductive health and overall well-being.

Even after very careful research and getting acceptable answers from your provider, your body may react negatively to the medication, or you may find yourself wanting to stop the medication. Stopping cold has worked for some or it may be a necessity. Whenever possible planning your transition off of the chosen medication can improve your body's response and align your body's hormones quicker than an abrupt stop.

Transitioning off Hormonal Birth Control

When deciding to transition off hormonal birth control, it is a similar process to when starting hormonal contraception. Our bodies take time to release the medication in our bodies, determine what hormones need to be made, and regulate the hormones now that medication has stopped. For those on the pill or mini pill, it could take 3-6 months or longer for your body to regulate. If prevention was a side benefit, be aware that the symptoms that initially plagued you prior to starting the medication, could return and be worse than before starting the medication. For those on long-term methods like the injection or implant, you'll also need time and support for your cycle to return and regulate. According to Pfizer, the manufacturer of Depo-Provera, it could take up to 18 months from the last injection for fertility to return. To minimize the body's shock when transitioning off the medication, begin supporting the body with nutrient dense foods, develop a sleep routine that includes 7-9 hours of sleep, start a self-care routine, and add 10-30 minutes of low to medium intensity exercise into your day about 3-6 months before stopping the medication.

Medications, estrogen, and many other hormones, toxins, vitamins, and nutrients are filtered out, produced, and/or regulated in the liver. A great way to support your liver is to stay hydrated. It is recommended that adults drink at least 64 ounces of water daily. I prefer the advice of drinking 1/2 your own body weight in ounces instead because 64 ounces of water might not be enough for your body. If it is warm, you are exercising, or sweating more than your typical amount, increase your intake of water. To easily know if you are properly hydrated, take a look at your urine. Urine in a hydrated body will be a very light-yellow color. Besides water, eating green leafy vegetables and high fiber foods help support the liver and move the excess toxins out of your body through the colon.

Nutrition plays a huge role in keeping our hormones aligned and our body feeling its best. While organic foods are ideal, I know they can be pricey. If organic is outside your budget limits, no worries! Just be sure to wash your fruits and veggies thoroughly to remove any pesticide residue. You can even use fruit and veggie wash to give them an extra good clean.

When it comes to meat, dairy, and fish, organic options are recommended because conventionally raised animals are often given hormones to make them grow faster. These hormones can end up in the meat, dairy, and fish we eat. Conventional animals are also typically fed genetically modified foods, which may contribute to inflammation in our bodies and hormonal imbalances. However, if organic is unavailable or outside your grocery budget, conventional animal products are still a great way to get the protein and nutrients your body needs.

I heard some great advise several years ago and I have been using it ever since on how to consume foods that give your body nutrients and help with maximum efficiency. Aim to eat foods in a particular order: fiber-rich veggies first, then protein and healthy fats, and finally carbs. Load up on fiber superstars like broccoli, spinach, brussels sprouts, and green peas. Then, get your protein from either plant or animal sources - aim for about 1 gram per pound of your body weight consumed over the course of the day. Some recommendations suggest eating around 30% of protein at each meal and 10-15% of protein at snacks. This is especially successful for those in peri-menopause at minimizing symptoms of weight gain. Awesome protein options include eggs, chicken, fish, tofu, lentils, and more. While I sometimes encounter skepticism about dietary fats, they are actually essential nutrients. Fats represent the most concentrated energy source in our food and play a crucial role in hormone production. Not all fats are identical; the body metabolizes different types of fat uniquely. To optimize nutrition, consider incorporating healthy fats like those found in avocados, olive oil, and coconut oil. When it comes to carbohydrates (carbs), stick to the low-glycemic kind as much as you can. These take longer to digest, so they won't spike your blood sugar or give you a sugar high. Think, whole grains, legumes,

> Fats represent the most concentrated energy source in our food and play a crucial role in hormone production.

nuts, seeds, quinoa, wild rice, oats, and berries. High-glycemic carbs like white bread, pasta, potatoes, and baked goods can mess with your hormones and fertility, so enjoy them sparingly. Within an hour after eating try and move your body for at least 10 minutes. This helps burn excess glucose in the blood stream before the meal is broken down, reducing blood sugar spikes.

Nurturing your body with nutrient-dense foods and keeping stress low are key for minimal symptoms involving your reproductive health. Chronic stress raises cortisol levels, inflammation, and fat accumulation which can disrupt other hormones like progesterone and estrogen. So be kind to yourself - your reproductive system and overall well-being will thank you!

Now that we've explored the diverse range of contraception methods available, you've gained valuable insights into their effects, considerations, and transition strategies. Remember that contraceptive choices are deeply personal decisions that should be made in partnership with healthcare professionals, seriously considering your unique needs, lifestyle, and well-being goals.

Throughout this book, we've journeyed together through the intricate dance of your hormones, the wisdom of your cyclic nature, and the powerful connection between your body, mind, and natural rhythms. You've learned that your menstrual cycle isn't just a monthly visitor – it's your personal superpower, influencing everything from your energy levels to your creativity, from your physical capabilities to your emotional intelligence.

Remember the cycle perspective activity you completed at the beginning of this book? Now it's time to revisit those same questions with fresh eyes and new understanding. As you compare your answers from then to now, you might be surprised to discover just how much your relationship with your cycle has evolved. This reflection is a powerful reminder of the knowledge you've gained and the mindset shifts you've experienced.

Now comes the exciting part: putting all this knowledge into practice! In the following pages, you'll find three months of detailed tracking sheets, engaging activities, and thoughtful journal prompts designed to help you discover your unique patterns and rhythms. Think of these tools as your personal laboratory for exploration and self-discovery. As you track, reflect, and engage with these activities, you'll begin to recognize the subtle shifts in your energy, mood, and capabilities throughout your cycle.

Remember, this isn't about perfection – it's about curiosity, self-discovery, and growing more confident in your body's wisdom with each passing cycle. Let's turn the page and start transforming this knowledge into practical, everyday magic. Your journey of living in harmony with your cycle begins now!

Summary:

- There are many types of preventative options available
- Become an advocate and give informed consent for your health and well-being
- Ask questions about your options, side effects both short and long term, and what happens if you experience severely negative side effects
- How to transition off hormonal birth control

My Cycle Perspective: After Our Journey

Date: _____

How I Now View My Cycle

What three words come to mind when you think about your cycle?

1. _____

2. _____

3. _____

Updated Pros & Cons of My Cycle

Pros (What I Like/Appreciate):

1. _____

2. _____

3. _____

Cons (What I've Learned to Navigate):

1. _____

2. _____

3. _____

Reflection Questions:

- How has your understanding of your cycle changed?

_____

_____

- What's the most valuable thing you've learned?

_____

_____

- How do you plan to use this knowledge in your daily life?

_____

_____

Dominate Your Period

CYCLE TRACKERS
AND ACTIVITIES

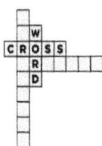

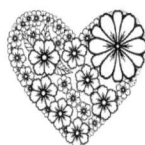

This section offers three months of guided period tracking, complete with self-care sheets tailored to each cycle phase, suggested activities, and reflective questions unique to each month. Building on the foundational knowledge shared earlier, these tools invite you to observe patterns, nurture your well-being, and align your actions with the natural rhythms of your body. Use this space as a personal guide to deepen your understanding and appreciation of your unique cycle.

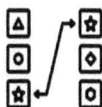

MAZE

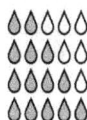

SECTION INCLUDES:

- **Emotion Wheel:** Scan the QR code to find out how to complete this activity and use the emotion colors with the period tracker sheets.
- **Tracker:** There are three trackers in this section to start getting into the habit of tracking. Refer to the Cycle Compass chapter for how to start.
- **Self-Care Boards:** List what self-care you will do during that particular month and phase. Get creative.
- **Phase Questions:** Reflective questions per phase each month.
- **Activities:** Are cycle aligned for each phase with answer keys.

The Emotion Wheel

To color in the wheel, start with the pieces in the middle. Pick a color for each triangular center wedge, "Sad, Mad, Scared, Joyful, Powerful, Peaceful". Each of these colors will be the brightest color on the wheel. Once a color is decided for each of those, choose a slightly less bright shade of the same color for the six emotions attached to the center triangular color. Once this is complete, decide on a very light shade of each chosen color for the final 12 spaces connected to the center triangular piece.

Example: Joyful is bright yellow, the second segment of 6 spaces that includes "Excited" is a sunshine yellow, the third section of 12 spaces including "Amused" is a pale yellow.

To view a coloring demo of the Emotion Wheel, please visit XX Strong's YouTube Channel or scan the QR Code that will take you directly there.

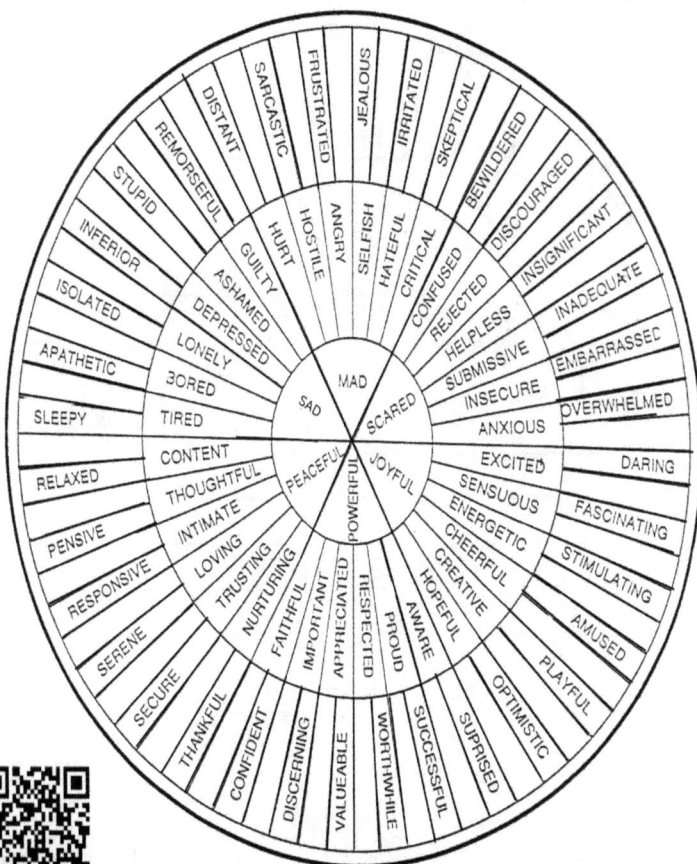

Developed by Dr. Gloria Wilcox   139

Dominate Your Period

Unleash Your Superpowers!

Day	1	2	3	4	5	6	7	8	9	10	11	12	13	14	15	16	17	18	19	20	21	22	23	24	25	26	27	28	29	30	31	32	33	34	35	36	37	38	39	40
Date																																								
Moon																																								
Flow																																								
Emotion																																								
Compete																																								
Notes																																								

Monthly Intentions

The first few days of your period is the perfect time to set intentions for the month. It is suportive of new beginnings and fresh starts. Write down your hopes, dreams, and goals using "I will or I am" statements

SELF CARE BOARD

List 4 self care tasks you will do this month
during the 9-18 days of luteal.

—PHASE DATE:

LUTEAL

Pedicure

Luteal Phase Questions

In the boxes below or on a separate paper write the answers to these questions or create your own reflective questions that start with "what".

What went well this month?

What didn't go as planned?

What do I want to continue doing?

What do I want to release or stop doing?

What felt overwhelming or stressful?

What brought me joy?

What is my focus next month?

What small change could make a difference?

What resources or support are needed?

What's one thing that I'm excited to start or try?

END the STIGMA

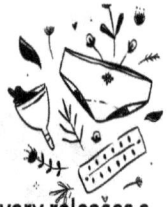

1. Menarche

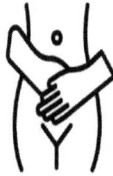

2. Ovulation

3. Mindset

4. Period Underwear

5. Spotting

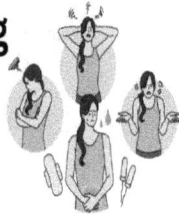

6. Ovum

7. Anovulation

8. REDs

9. Uterus

10. PMS

Match the Correct Answers

A. The process where an ovary releases a mature egg.

B. A mature egg that is released from the ovary at ovulation.

C. Minimal bleeding. Can be experienced around ovulation, beginning of menstruation, or end of menstruation.

D. A combination of physical and emotional symptoms that appear from three to ten days before a period arrives.

E. Strong upside-down pear-shaped organ used to carry and grow a baby or babies

F. An energy imbalance leading to impaired physiological function of multiple organ systems & involves any one or more of the following three components that are often interrelated: low energy availability, menstrual dysfunction, & low bone mineral density.

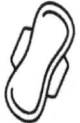

G. A collection of underlying beliefs, attitudes, and mental habits

H. A female's first menstrual period, usually occurring during puberty

I. Specially made underwear to be worn during menstruation.

J. When an egg fails to be released at ovulation during a cycle.

SELF CARE BOARD

List 4 self care tasks you will do this month
during the 3-7 days of menstruation.

PHASE DATE:

MENSTRUAL ❄

- Reading
-
-
-
-

Menstrual Phase Questions

In the boxes below or on a separate paper refer to the answers from the Luteal phase then write the answers to these questions.

Why did they go well?

Why didn't it go as planned?

Why do I want to continue?

Why do I want to release or stop doing?

Why did it feel overwhelming or stressful?

Why was there joy?

Why is it my focus for next month?

Why could a small change make a difference?

Why are the resources or support needed?

Why am I excited?

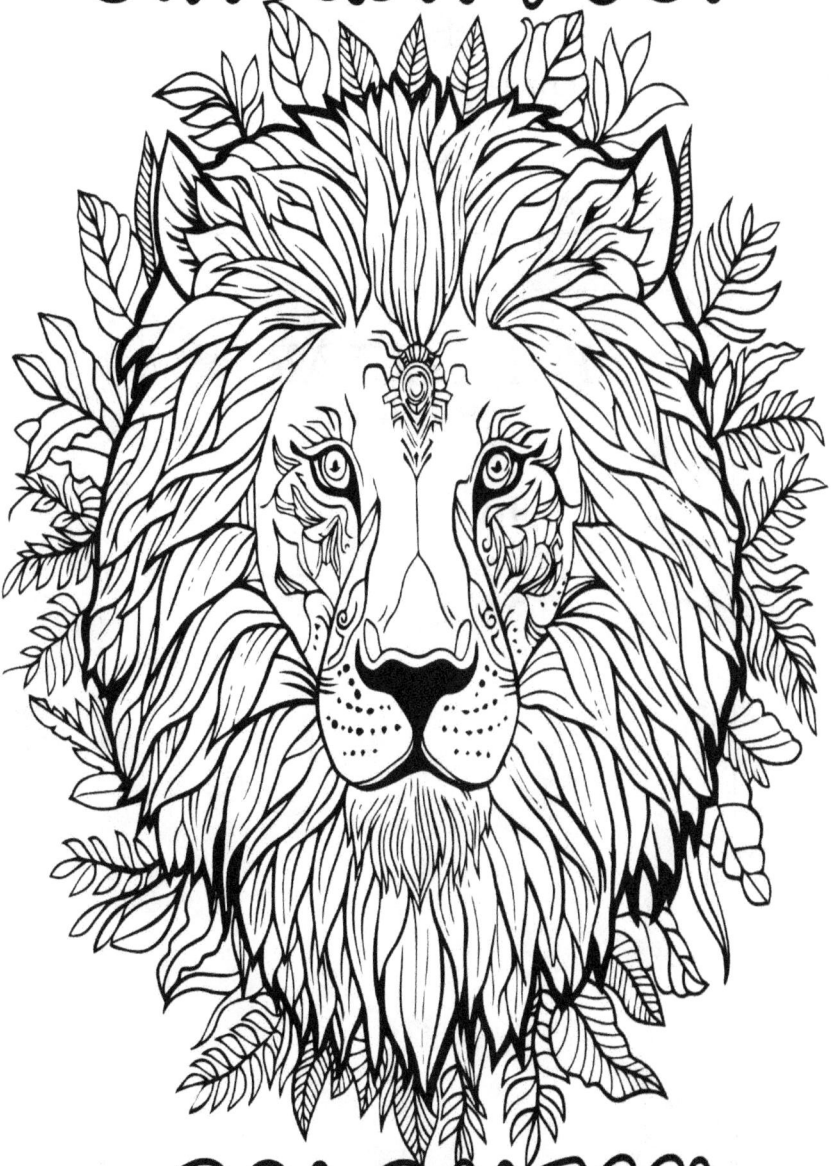

Unleash Your
BOLDNESS!

SELF CARE BOARD

List 4 self care tasks you will do this month
during the days of follicular.

PHASE DATE:

FOLLICULAR

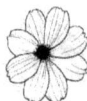

Hot/Cold Plunge

Follicular Phase Questions

In the boxes below or on a separate paper refer to the answers from the Luteal/Menstrual phases then write the answers to these questions.

How is the outcome maintained?

How can I improve the outcome?

How am I going to continue incorporating?

How do I let go?

How do I reduce overwhelm or stress?

How do I maintain joy?

How will the plan work?

How do I make the small change?

How do I receive the resources or support needed?

How do I start?

DOMINATE YOUR PERIOD

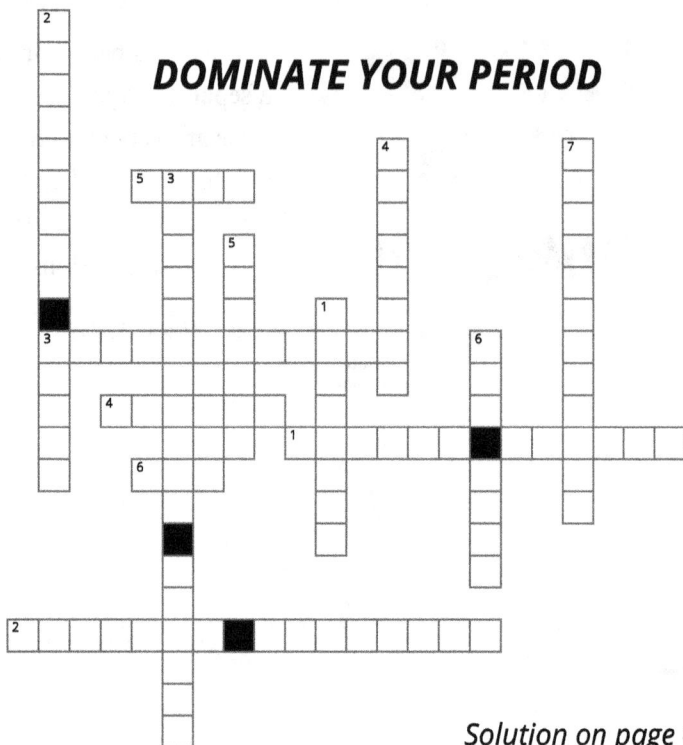

Solution on page #179

Across:

1. A temporary structure that forms in the ovary after an egg is released during ovulation.

2. Items used to help manage menstrual flow and maintain cleanliness during menstruation including pads, tampons, menstrual cups, and period underwear.

3. Hormone produced throughout a lifetime by adrenal glands, the corpus luteum considered the calming hormone.

4. A muscular canal that links the uterus to the vagina.

5. Fertility Education and Medical Management is an education and prevention based reproductive health program.

6. Essential nutrient that the body needs for energy, organ protection, and hormone production.

Down:

1. Chemical messengers that tell the body what to do.

2. Shedding of the endometrial lining signalling the beginning of a new cycle.

3. Lining of the uterus that grows during the follicular phase and sheds at menstruation.

4. A hormone produced by several sources throughout a lifetime.

5. An essential nutrient that helps build and repair tissues in our body.

6. Technology that removes the negative emotional response to a specific memory of a past event or fear

7. type of nutrient found in many foods that provide the body with energy. They come in different forms including sugars, starches, and fibers.

SELF CARE BOARD

List 4 self care tasks you will do this month
during the 3-4 days of ovulation.

OVULATION ☀

Dance

Ovulation Phase

Go do the answers to the questions from Follicular phase.

LET'S DO this

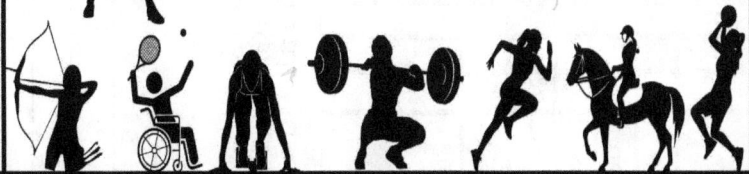

GET OUT AND MOVE...

Unleash Your Super Powers

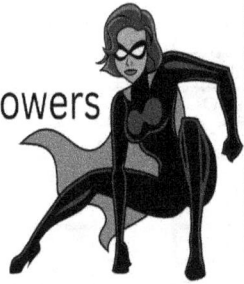

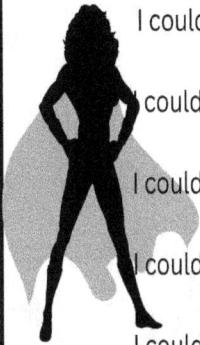

I could... _____

I could... _____

I could... _____

I could... _____

I could... _____

I will... _____

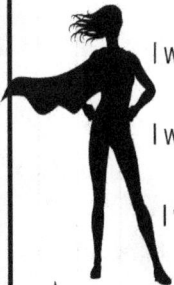

I will.. _____

I will... _____

I will... _____

Day	1	2	3	4	5	6	7	8	9	10	11	12	13	14	15	16	17	18	19	20	21	22	23	24	25	26	27	28	29	30	31	32	33	34	35	36	37	38	39	40
Date																																								
Moon																																								
Flow																																								
Emotion																																								
Compete																																								
Notes																																								

Monthly Intentions

The first few days of your period is the perfect time to set intentions for the month. It is suportive of new beginnings and fresh starts. Write down your hopes, dreams, and goals using "I will or I am" statements

SELF CARE BOARD

List 4 self care tasks you will do this month
during the 9-18 days of luteal.

PHASE DATE:

LUTEAL

- Pedicure

Luteal Phase Questions

In the boxes below or on a separate paper write the answers to these questions or create your own reflective questions that start with "what".

What went well this month?

What didn't go as planned?

What do I want to continue doing?

What do I want to release or stop doing?

What felt overwhelming or stressful?

What brought me joy?

What is my focus next month?

What small change could make a difference?

What resources or support are needed?

What's one thing that I'm excited to start or try?

Schulte Tables for Focus & Awareness

Reaction Training:

Start at 1 and touch the numbers in ascending or descending order as quickly as possible.

Scan the table horizontally and vertically to find all the numbers in order as quickly as possible

Time yourself or have a coach time you to track progress.

Focus and Awareness:

Instead of touching the numbers, verbally call out each number as you find it.

Increase the challenge by calling out the next number but touching the previous one (e.g., say "2" but touch "1").

Cognitive Flexibility:

Try finding the numbers or letters in a reverse order (25 to 1) or (Z to A).

Alternatively, you can find odd numbers first and then even numbers.

Game Options:

Find Odd / Even numbers   Name the sporting equipment

Name the letters   Create your own tables

Challenge team members and friends   Play for speed & accuracy

Skip by multiples. 2s, 3s, 4s, 4s, 5s, and so on through the 10 x 10 tables

Memorize rows and columns; see how many you can recite without error

MAKE IT FUN AND CHALLENGING!

4	22	15	9	11
13	1	21	16	5
20	8	3	17	14
24	7	19	10	6
18	12	2	23	25

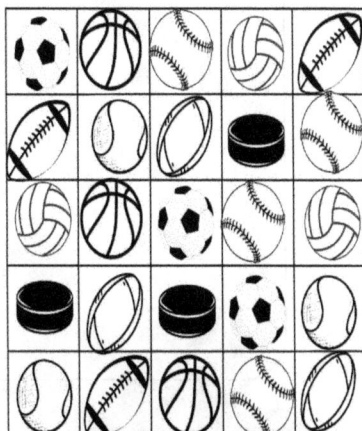

SELF CARE BOARD

List 4 self care tasks you will do this month
during the 3-7 days of menstruation.

PHASE DATE:

MENSTRUAL ❄

- ⬤ Reading
- ⬤
- ⬤
- ⬤
- ⬤

Menstrual Phase Questions

In the boxes below or on a separate paper refer to the answers from the Luteal phase then write the answers to these questions.

Why did they go well?

Why didn't it go as planned?

Why do I want to continue?

Why do I want to release or stop doing?

Why did it feel overwhelming or stressful?

Why was there joy?

Why is it my focus for next month?

Why could a small change make a difference?

Why are the resources or support needed?

Why am I excited?

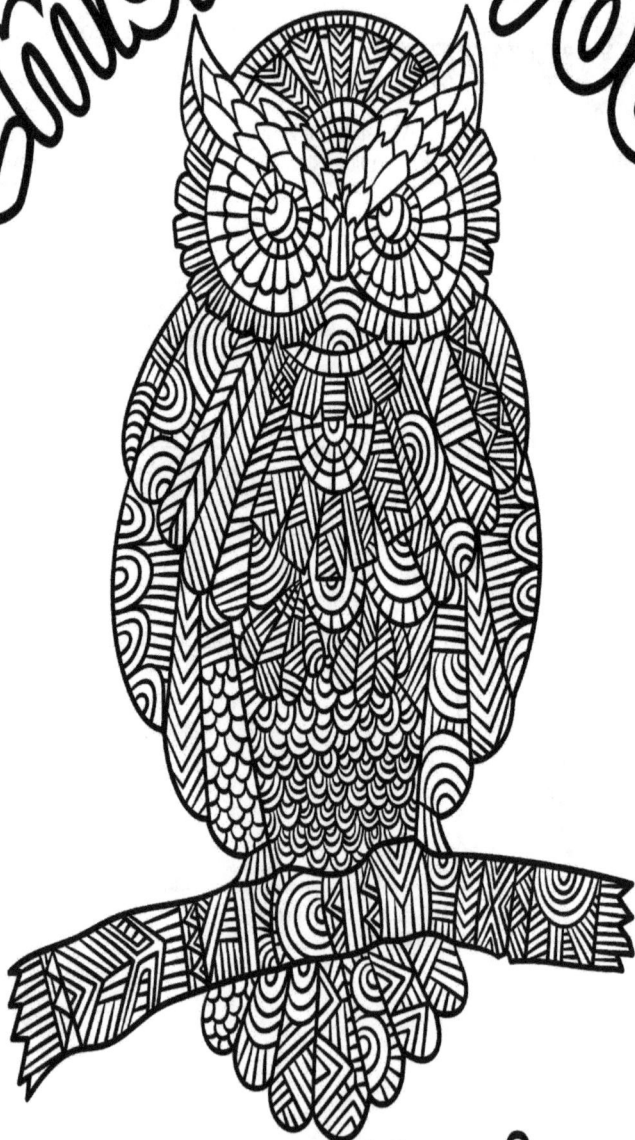

Embrace your Inner Wisdom!

SELF CARE BOARD

List 4 self care tasks you will do this month
during the days of follicular.

PHASE DATE:

FOLLICULAR

◯ Hot/Cold Plunge

◯

◯

◯

◯

Follicular Phase Questions

In the boxes below or on a separate paper refer to the answers from the Luteal/Menstrual phases then write the answers to these questions.

How is the outcome maintained?

How can I improve the outcome?

How am I going to continue incorporating?

How do I let go?

How do I reduce overwhelm or stress?

How do I maintain joy?

How will the plan work ?

How do I make the small change?

How do I receive the resources or support needed?

How do I start?

SYSTEMS & CHOICES

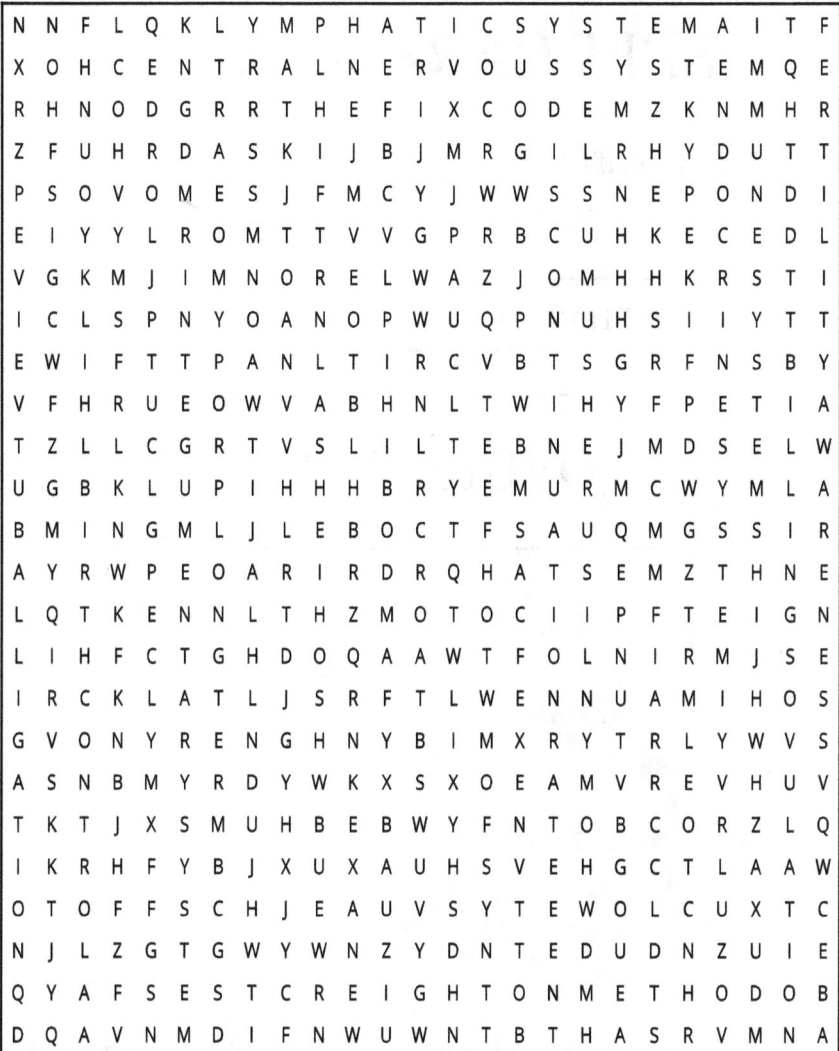

```
N N F L Q K L Y M P H A T I C S Y S T E M A I T F
X O H C E N T R A L N E R V O U S S Y S T E M Q E
R H N O D G R R T H E F I X C O D E M Z K N M H R
Z F U H R D A S K I J B J M R G I L R H Y D U T T
P S O V O M E S J F M C Y J W W S S N E P O N D I
E I Y Y L R O M T T V V G P R B C U H K E C E D L
V G K M J I M N O R E L W A Z J O M H H K R S T I
I C L S P N Y O A N O P W U Q P N U H S I I Y T T
E W I F T T P A N L T I R C V B T S G R F N S B Y
V F H R U E O W V A B H N L T W I H Y F P E T I A
T Z L L C G R T V S L I L T E B N E J M D S E L W
U G B K L U P I H H H B R Y E M U R M C W Y M L A
B M I N G M L J L E B O C T F S A U Q M G S S I R
A Y R W P E O A R I R D R Q H A T S E M Z T H N E
L Q T K E N N L T H Z M O T O C I I P F T E I G N
L I H F C T G H D O Q A A W T F O L N I R M J S E
I R C K L A T L J S R F T L W E N N U A M I H O S
G V O N Y R E N G H N Y B I M X R Y T R L Y W V S
A S N B M Y R D Y W K X S X O E A M V R E V H U V
T K T J X S M U H B E B W Y F N T O B C O R Z L Q
I K R H F Y B J X U X A U H S V E H G C T L A A W
O T O F F S C H J E A U V S Y T E W O L C U X T C
N J L Z G T G W Y W N Z Y D N T E D U D N Z U I E
Q Y A F S E S T C R E I G H T O N M E T H O D O B
D Q A V N M D I F N W U W N T B T H A S R V M N A
```

HORMONAL BIRTH CONTROL

CREIGHTON METHOD

FERTILITY AWARENESS

STERILIZATION

SHORT TERM BC

CENTRAL NERVOUS SYSTEM

INTEGUMENTARY SYSTEM

LONG TERM BC

BIRTH CONTROL

DISCONTINUATION RATE

SYMPTO-THERMAL METHOD

THE FIX CODE

GASTROINTESTINAL

LYMPHATIC SYSTEM

BILLINGS OVULATION

MONTHLY FAILURE RATE

TUBAL LIGATION

NON HORMONAL BC

CIRCULATORY SYSTEM

IMMUNE SYSTEM

ENDOCRINE SYSTEM

Solution on page #179

SELF CARE BOARD

List 4 self care tasks you will do this month
during the 3-4 days of ovulation.

—PHASE DATE:

OVULATION

Dance

Ovulation Phase

Go do the answers to the questions from Follicular phase.

LET'S DO this

Reflex Reaction Activity
Action Words

Reflex Reaction activities enhance your quick-thinking and decision-making skills with fun and challenging words, numbers, and related images!

These activities are designed to be engaging and fun while secretly training crucial skills such as:

Response Inhibition Visual Scanning
Sport-Specific Focus Motor Planning
Predictive Skills Numerical processing

Quick Decision-Making Visual Discrimination
Visual Recognition Visual Perception

The following contains distinct activities designed to improve different aspects of an athlete's cognitive and reactive skills.

CIRCLE then DO the ACTION Words   CROSS OUT the NON-ACTION Words

JUMP	SPIN	SKIP	SQUAT	THROW	Duck	Punch	RUN	HOP	COACH
THROW	Punch	Duck	HOP	COURT	PHASE	JUMP	CALL	POINT	SPIN
F.I.X.	CODE	HOP	RUN	BENCH	Punch	HOP	FLOOR	TIME	RUN
PADS	RUN	FUN	JUMP	CRAMPS	SQUAT	SPIN	Punch	CANAL	FIELD
SQUAT	Punch	CANAL	Duck	HOP	FAN	RUN	JUMP	WIN	THROW
THROW	Duck	HOP	BALL	FUN	Punch	TRACK	POOL	F.I.X.	CODE
HOP	CYCLE	PADS	RUN	LOSE	THROW	HYPE	PADS	HOP	JUMP
JUMP	THROW	RUN	GLOVE	Duck	BAR	Punch	PHONE	RUN	BALL
CYCLE	Punch	CODE	JUMP	HOP	F.I.X.	CODE	BEAM	Duck	SAFE
Duck	SPIN	TOOL	HOP	Phase	Punch	JUMP	PHASE	SQUAT	SPIN
HOP	Punch	JUMP	YARD	RUN	HOP	Duck	GREEN	HOP	STOP

Day	1	2	3	4	5	6	7	8	9	10	11	12	13	14	15	16	17	18	19	20	21	22	23	24	25	26	27	28	29	30	31	32	33	34	35	36	37	38	39	40
Date																																								
Moon																																								
Flow																																								
Emotion																																								
Compete																																								
Notes																																								

Monthly Intentions

The first few days of your period is the perfect time to set intentions for the month. It is suportive of new beginnings and fresh starts. Write down your hopes, dreams, and goals using "I will or I am" statements

SELF CARE BOARD

List 4 self care tasks you will do this month
during the 9-18 days of luteal.

—PHASE DATE:

LUTEAL

Pedicure

Luteal Phase Questions

In the boxes below or on a separate paper write the answers to these questions or create your own reflective questions that start with "what".

What went well this month?

What didn't go as planned?

What do I want to continue doing?

What do I want to release or stop doing?

What felt overwhelming or stressful?

What brought me joy?

What is my focus next month?

What small change could make a difference?

What resources or support are needed?

What's one thing that I'm excited to start or try?

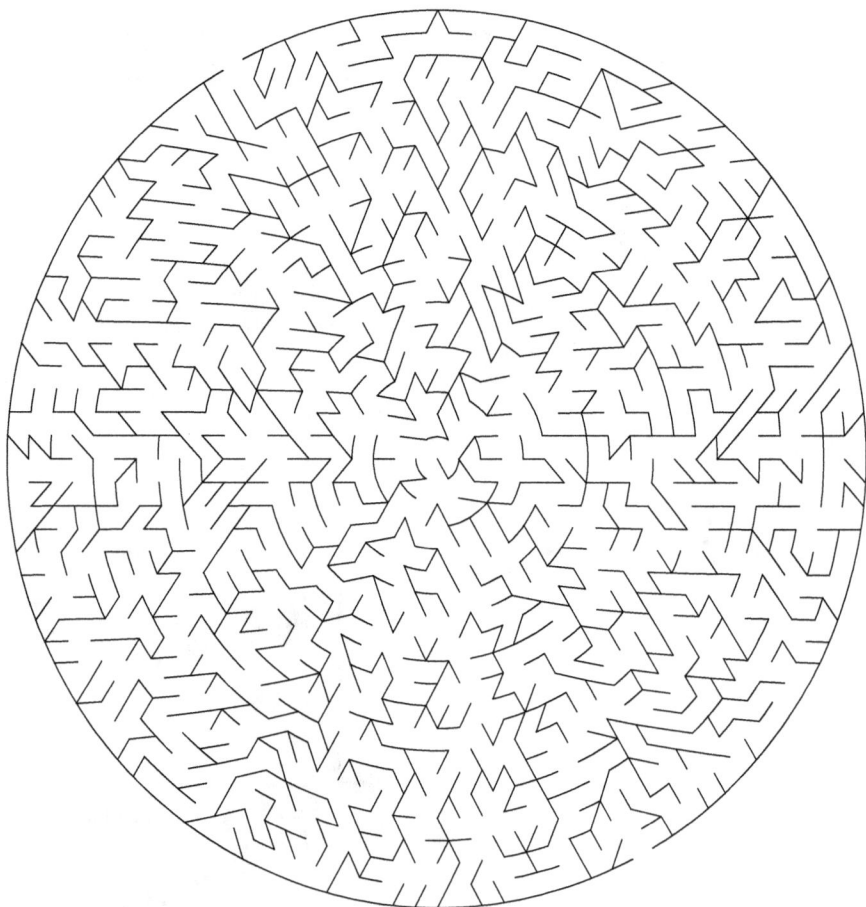

Solution on page #180

SELF CARE BOARD

List 4 self care tasks you will do this month
during the 3-7 days of menstruation.

—————PHASE DATE: —————

MENSTRUAL ❄️

- Reading
-
-
-
-

Menstrual Phase Questions

In the boxes below or on a separate paper refer to the answers from the Luteal phase then write the answers to these questions.

Why did they go well?

Why didn't it go as planned?

Why do I want to continue?

Why do I want to release or stop doing?

Why did it feel overwhelming or stressful?

Why was there joy?

Why is it my focus for next month?

Why could a small change make a difference?

Why are the resources or support needed?

Why am I excited?

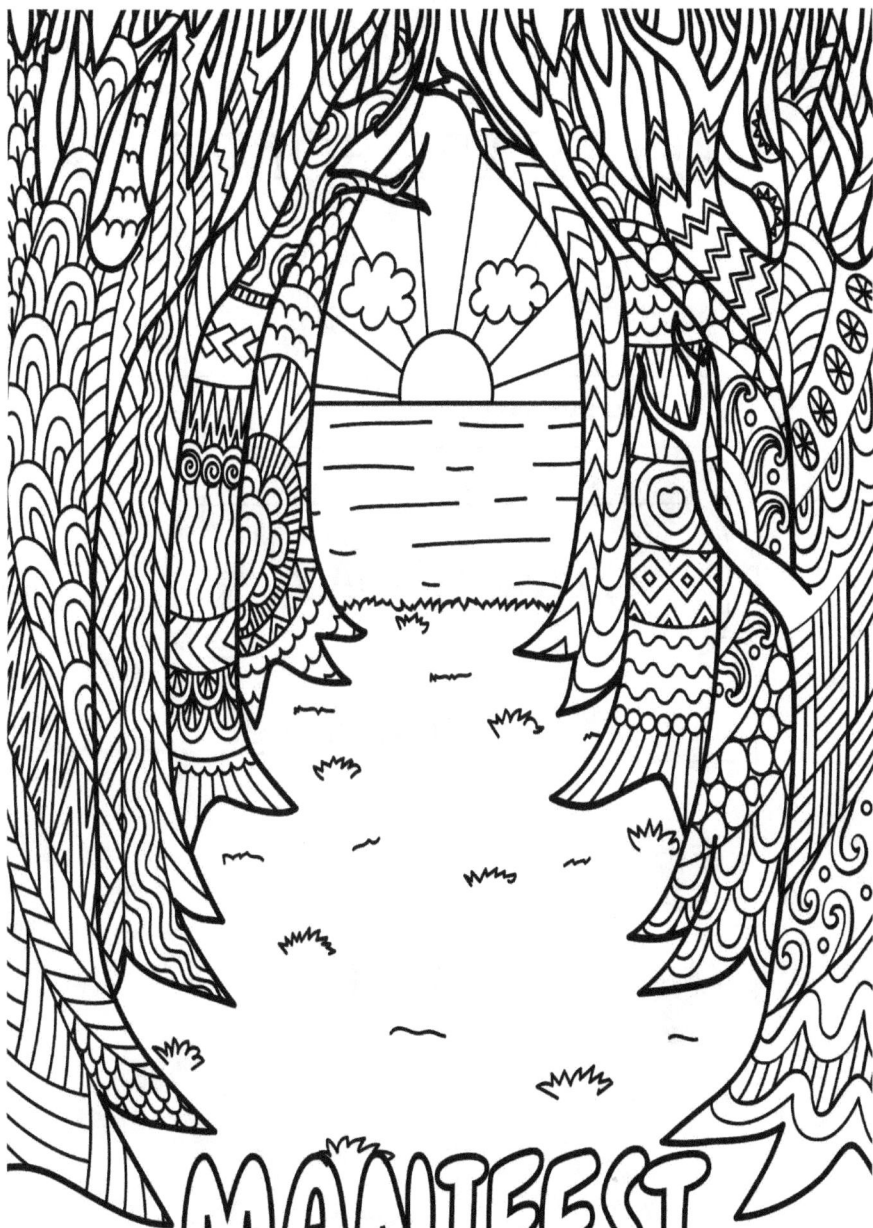

MANIFEST YOUR DREAMS!

SELF CARE BOARD

List 4 self care tasks you will do this month
during the days of follicular.

PHASE DATE:

FOLLICULAR

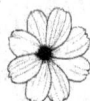

Hot/Cold Plunge

Follicular Phase Questions

In the boxes below or on a separate paper refer to the answers from the Luteal/Menstrual phases then write the answers to these questions.

How is the outcome maintained?

How can I improve the outcome?

How am I going to continue incorporating?

How do I let go?

How do I reduce overwhelm or stress?

How do I maintain joy?

How will the plan work ?

How do I make the small change?

How do I receive the resources or support needed?

How do I start?

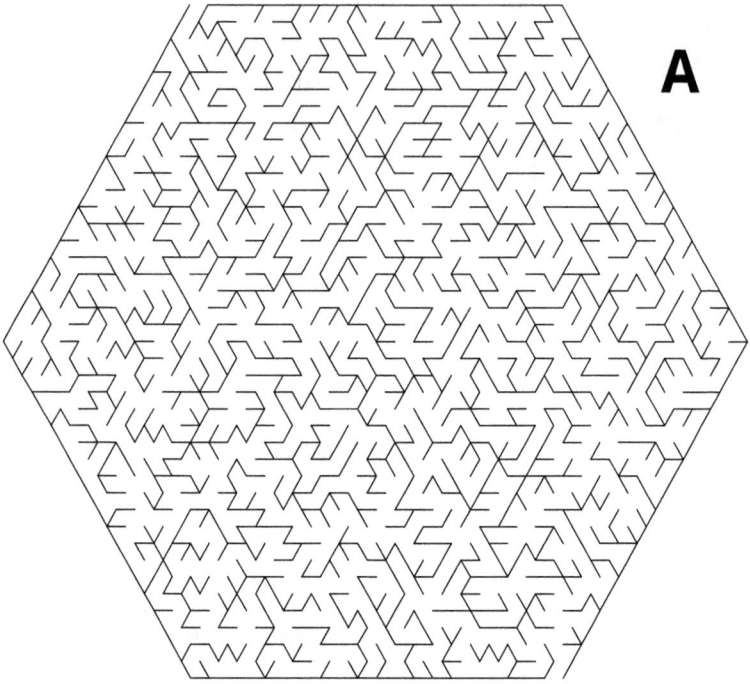

A

A

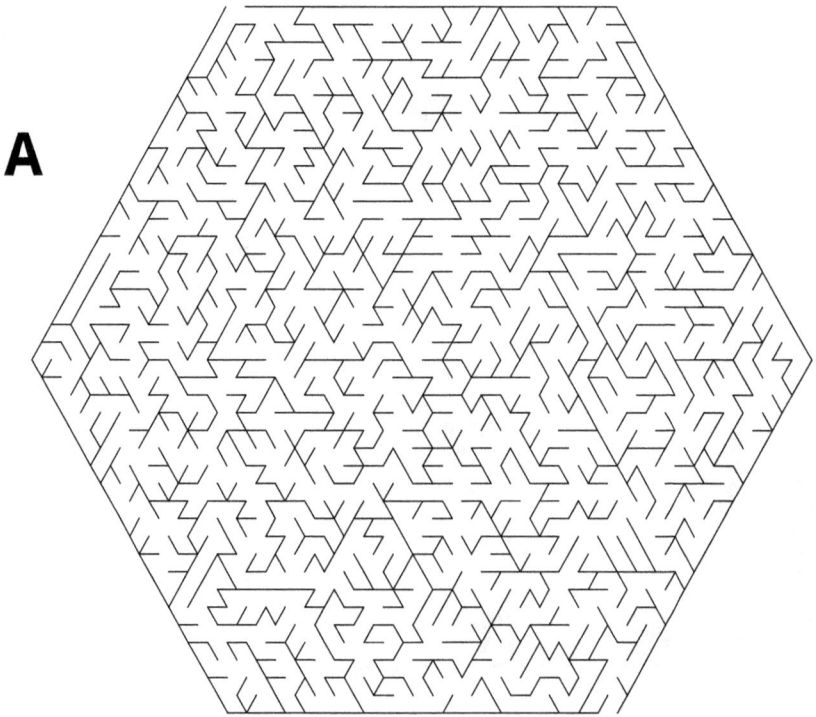

Solutions on page #180

SELF CARE BOARD

List 4 self care tasks you will do this month
during the 3-4 days of ovulation.

—PHASE DATE:

OVULATION

- ○ Dance
- ○
- ○
- ○
- ○

Ovulation Phase

Go do the answers to the questions from Follicular phase.

LET'S DO this

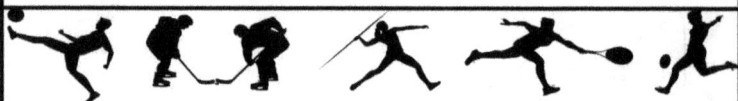

GET OUT AND MOVE...

Unleash Your Super Powers

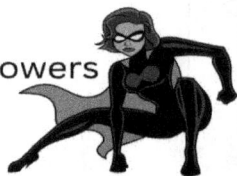

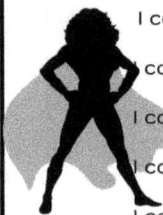

I could... _____

I could... _____

I could... _____

I could... _____

I could... _____

I will... _____

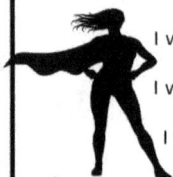

I will.. _____

I will... _____

I will... _____

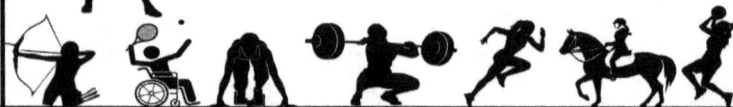

DOMINATE YOUR PERIOD

From page #150

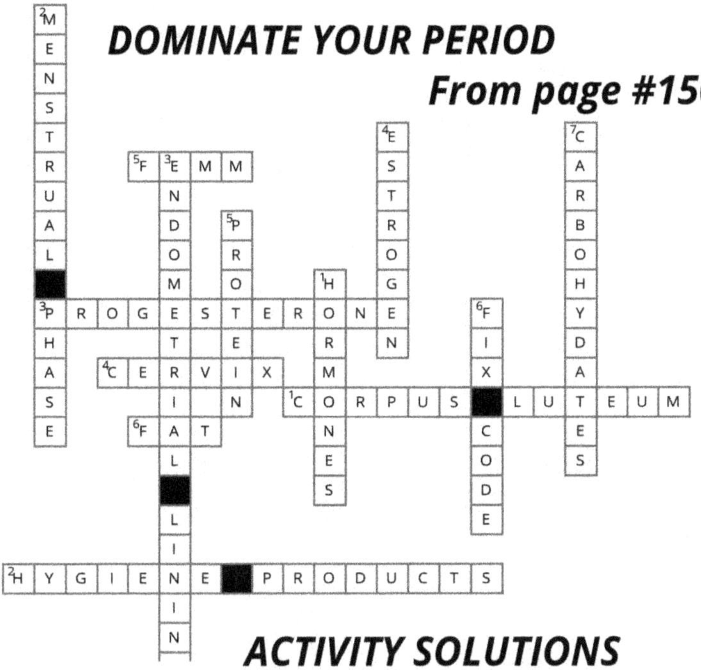

ACTIVITY SOLUTIONS

SYSTEMS & CHOICES

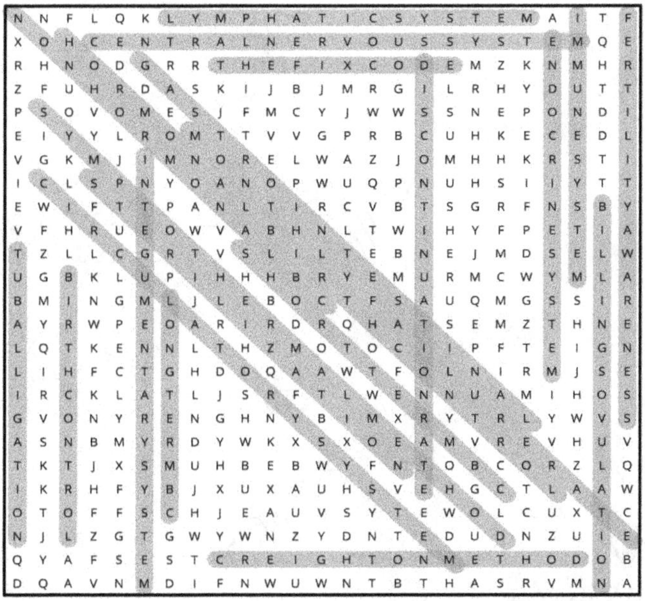

From page #163

ACTIVITY SOLUTIONS

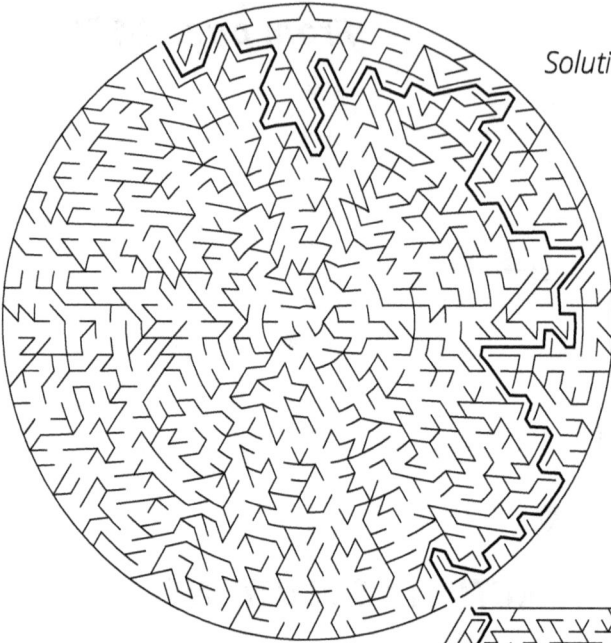

Solution from page 170

Solutions from page 176

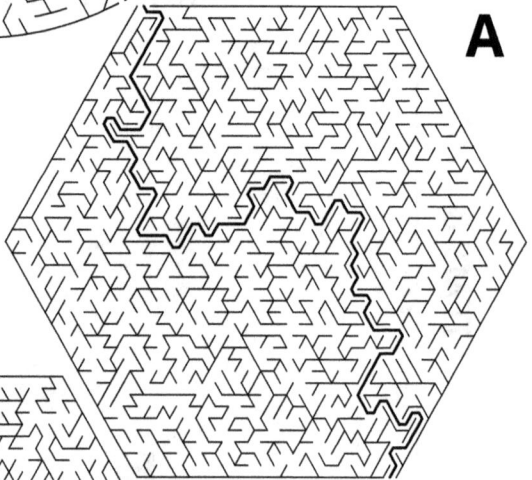

A

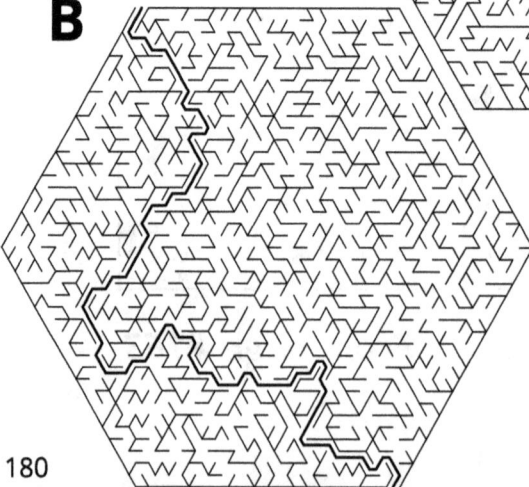

B

GLOSSARY

Anovulation: When an egg fails to be released at ovulation during a cycle.

Basal Body Temperature: Your body temperature when you are totally at rest for at least 3 hours of continuous sleep.

Billings Ovulation Method: A way to understand the menstrual cycle by observing changes in cervical mucus. It involves checking and recording the feel and appearance of mucus at the vaginal opening each day, helping to identify different phases of the cycle.

Biomarkers: The body's vital signs like cervical mucus, heart rate, blood pressure, and temperature. Observing these signs regularly enables recognition, accurate testing, and early treatment of possible health issues by medical providers.

Birth Control: Is the use of hormones or non-hormonal methods, devices, or medication to prevent pregnancy.

Bladder: A sac that holds urine until released when using the restroom.

Carbohydrates: Also known as carbs are a type of nutrient found in many foods that provide the body with energy. They come in different forms including sugars, starches, and fibers. The body breaks down carbohydrates into glucose which cells can use for fuel or store for later use. The breakdown into glucose varies depending on the composition of the nutrient. See Glycemic Index for more information.

Central Nervous System: Is your body's main control center, consisting of the brain and spinal cord. It processes information from your senses, controls your movements and thoughts, and manages important body functions like breathing.

Cervical Mucus: A fluid produced by glands in a woman's cervix that changes throughout her menstrual cycle. It acts as a natural sign of hormonal function in relation to health.

Cervical Position: Refers to the location and feel of the cervix, which changes throughout a woman's menstrual cycle. These changes in the cervix's height, firmness, and openness can indicate different stages of the cycle, including when a woman is about to ovulate.

Cervical Texture: Describes how the cervix feels to the touch, changing from firm to soft during a woman's menstrual cycle. This change in texture, along with position and openness, can help indicate fertile periods, with the cervix becoming softer and more velvety during ovulation.

Cervix: A muscular canal that links the uterus to the vagina. This organ allows for the passage of fluids between the uterine and vaginal cavities. It plays a vital role in the cycling of menstrual flow and the birth process itself.

Circulatory System: Is the body's network of blood vessels and the heart that moves blood throughout the body. It delivers oxygen and nutrients to all parts of the body and removes waste products, playing a crucial role in keeping us alive and healthy.

Corpus Luteum: A temporary structure that forms in the ovary after an egg is released during ovulation. It produces hormones like progesterone that prepare the uterus for a possible pregnancy and, if no pregnancy occurs, it breaks down, leading to menstruation.

Creighton Method: Relies upon the standardized observation and charting of biological markers that are essential to a woman's health and fertility. It is a standardized modification of the Billings Ovulation Method.

Cycle Length: The number of days between the first day of one menstrual period and the first day of the next. A typical cycle length is around 28 days, but it can vary from person to person and even from cycle to cycle in the same individual.

Discontinuation Rate: Approximate percentage of users who have stopped taking a particular medication for method related reasons within a 12 month time frame.

Emotion Wheel: A visual tool that helps people identify and understand different feelings they might experience. It organizes emotions into categories, starting with basic feelings in the center and expanding outward to more complex and specific emotions, helping people better recognize and express their emotional states.

Endocrine System: A network of glands that produce and release hormones into the bloodstream controlling various body functions like growth, metabolism, mood, and reproduction.

Endometrial Lining: Lining of the uterus that grows during the follicular phase and sheds at menstruation. This is also the place where an embryo attaches itself for nutrients during pregnancy.

Estrogen: A hormone produced by several sources throughout a lifetime. It is produced by the adrenal glands and adipose tissue before puberty as well as after menopause and by the ovaries during reproductive years. It is considered a growth hormone and a major player in the biological female reproductive system along with progesterone.

Estrous ('estrǝs): Menstrual cycles where the biological female animal goes through a similar process to biological female humans, however, absorbs the endometrial lining, the exception to this is dogs.

Fallopian Tubes: A pair of tubes that carries an egg (ovum) from the ovary to the uterus

Fat: An essential nutrient that the body needs for energy, organ protection, and hormone production. It comes in different types, including healthy fats found in foods like avocados and nuts, and less healthy fats found in some processed foods, with each type playing a different role in our health.

FEMM: Fertility Education and Medical Management is an education and prevention based reproductive health program.

Fertility Awareness: Method of understanding the different phases of a woman's menstrual cycle. It involves observing and recording natural body signs like temperature changes and cervical mucus to learn about the cycle's patterns and hormonal shifts.

Follicle: A small, fluid-filled sac in the ovary that contains a developing egg. Each month, several follicles start to grow, but usually only one becomes mature and releases its egg during ovulation.

Follicular Phase: The first part of the menstrual cycle, starting on the first day of menstruation. During this phase, follicles in the ovary grow and develop, preparing to release an egg, while the uterine lining begins to thicken.

Follicular Stimulating Hormone: Is produced and released by the pituitary gland located in the brain. It is responsible for triggering breast development and menstruation in puberty and regulating the menstrual cycle between puberty and menopause.

Gastrointestinal System: Also called the digestive system, is the group of organs that process food in your body. It includes organs like the stomach, intestines, and liver, which break down food, absorb nutrients, and remove waste.

Glycemic Index: A measure of how quickly a food containing carbohydrates raises a person's blood sugar levels. Foods with a high glycemic index cause a rapid spike in blood sugar, while those with a low glycemic index result in a slower, more gradual increase. This information can help people make healthier choices about the types of carbohydrates they consume.

Heavy Menstrual Flow: Also called menorrhagia, refers to periods that are unusually heavy or long-lasting. It's characterized by needing to change pads or tampons more than 5 times a day, a product change within an hour, passing large blood clots, or having periods that last longer than a week. Fluid loss is <25ml or having to change a menstrual cup more than one time per day. Blood color is typically red or dark red.

Hormonal Birth Control: Medications providing low levels of synthetic hormones to suppress natural hormonal activity in the body. They inhibit ovarian follicle development, attempt to prevent ovulation, thin the endometrial lining making it difficult for a fertilized egg to implant, and thicken cervical mucus, making it difficult for sperm to reach the uterus.

Hormones: Chemical messengers that tell the body what to do.

Hygiene Products: Items used to help manage menstrual flow and maintain cleanliness during menstruation including pads, tampons, menstrual cups, and period underwear.

Immune System: The body's defense network against harmful germs and substances. It includes special cells, tissues, and organs that work together to identify and fight off invaders like bacteria and viruses, helping to keep us healthy.

Informed Consent: Making health decisions after learning about and considering all the options and information available.

Integumentary System: The body's outer protective layer, primarily made up of the skin. It also includes hair, nails, and sweat glands, working together to protect the body from injury, regulating temperature, and sense the environment around us.

Light Menstrual Flow: Refers to periods that are unusually light in flow and very short. It's characterized by needing to change pads or tampons one to two times a day, it is sometimes seen at the beginning or end of the menstrual phase. Fluid loss is 5-15ml or 1/3 to 1/4 filled menstrual cup. Blood color can be brown, black, pink, red or dark red.

Long-Term Hormonal Contraceptives: Medications that are hormonal in nature and usually require medical approval. These methods are effective for several years and require medical professionals to insert and remove the method of contraceptive.

Luteal Phase: The second half of a menstrual cycle from ovulation until the day before menstruation.

Luteinizing Hormone: Is produced and released by the pituitary gland in the brain. It is responsible for triggering ovulation during reproductive years.

Lymphatic System: A network of vessels and tissues that helps remove waste and fight infections in the body. It works alongside the circulatory system, collecting excess fluid from tissues, filtering out harmful substances, and returning clean fluid back to the bloodstream.

Medium Menstrual Flow: Refers to periods that are consistent in flow with a bright red color. It's characterized by needing to change pads or tampons 3-4 times. Fluid loss is 15-25ml or 1/2 to almost full menstrual cup.

Menarche: Term for a biological females first menstrual period, usually occurring during puberty. It marks the beginning of the reproductive years and typically happens between ages 10 and 15, with the average around 12-13 years of age, though the exact timing can vary for everyone.

Menstrual Cup/Disc: A flexible, round device inserted into the vagina to collect menstrual flow. It sits higher than a menstrual cup, fitting in the vaginal fornix near the cervix, and can be worn for up to 12 hours, including during physical activities

Menstrual Cycle: A natural monthly hormonal routine the XX chromosome (biological female) body uses to maintain the overall health of 11 bodily systems using the rise and fall of 12 specific hormones ending in a shedding of the endometrial lining.

Menstrual Dysfunction: Problems or irregularities with a person's menstrual cycle. This can include issues like irregular periods, unusually heavy or light flow, severe cramps, or the absence of periods, which may indicate underlying health concerns or hormonal imbalances.

Menstruation/Menstrual Phase/Menses: An important indicator of health for the biological female during reproductive years. It involves the uterus shedding the endometrial lining, signaling the beginning of a new cycle. The nature of the blood flow can provide clues about hormone levels and overall health.

Mindset: A collection of underlying beliefs, attitudes, and mental habits we hold about ourselves and shapes how we approach challenges, embrace growth, and perceive potential.

Monthly Failure Rate: Approximate percentage of users who get pregnant using a particular contraceptive, with either perfect or typical use.

Musculoskeletal System: The body's framework of bones, muscles, and connective tissues. It provides structure, support, and allows movement, while also protecting internal organs and storing minerals essential for bodily functions.

Non-Hormonal Birth Control: A preventative method that allows the body to maintain natural levels of hormonal activity while attempting to prevent an ovulated egg reaching sperm.

Ovaries: A pair of oval sacs that hold all ovarian follicles prior to ovulation. Also generates the corpus luteum after ovulation.

Ovulation: The process where an ovary releases a mature egg.

Ovulation Phase: The time in a cycle where cervical mucus feels or looks like lotion or like clear jelly, the luteinizing hormone rises, an ovary releases a mature ovum to be swept into a fallopian tube, and the remaining follicular shell becomes the corpus luteum.

Ovum: A mature egg that is released from the ovary at ovulation.

Perineum: A small area of skin with many nerve endings between the vaginal opening and the rectum

Period Underwear: Specially made underwear to be worn during menstruation.

Premenstrual Dysphoric Disorder (PMDD): A more serious form of premenstrual syndrome involving symptoms of PMS, with severe episodes of anxiety, depression, or both, suicidal ideologies, pain that renders the person unable to move three to 14 days before a period arrives.

Premenstrual Syndrome (PMS): A combination of physical and emotional symptoms that appear from three to ten days before a period arrives.

Progesterone: A hormone produced by several sources throughout a lifetime. It is produced by the adrenal glands before puberty as well as after menopause and by the corpus luteum in the ovaries during reproductive years. It is considered the calming hormone and is a major player in the biological female reproductive system along with it's partner estrogen.

Protein: An essential nutrient that helps build and repair tissues in our body. It's found in foods like meat, eggs, beans, and nuts, and is important for making muscles, bones, skin, and blood, as well as for producing enzymes and hormones

Rectum: Exterior opening to the large intestines where solid waste is removed from the body.

Relative Energy Deficiency In Sports (RED-S): A condition in which energy imbalance leads to impaired physiological function of multiple organ systems and involves any one or more of the following three components that are often interrelated: low energy availability, menstrual dysfunction, and low bone mineral density.

Reproductive System: A group of organs in the body that are involved in human development and growth. In females, it includes the ovaries, uterus, and vagina, while in males it includes the testicles and penis, with each part playing a specific role in the body's changes during puberty and adulthood.

Reproductive Years: Refer to the time in a person's life when their body is capable of pregnancy. For most women, this period starts with their first menstrual period during puberty and ends with menopause, typically spanning from the early teens to around age 50.

Respiratory System: Is the group of organs that help us breathe. It includes the nose, throat, lungs, and airways, working together to bring oxygen into our body when we inhale and remove carbon dioxide when we exhale.

Sanitary pads: A flat piece of cotton or cotton blend material attached to a plastic bottom with an open weaved layer on top to trap and hold menstrual fluid

Sexually Transmitted Illness: Infections that can spread from person to person during sexual contact. They are caused by bacteria, viruses, or parasites and can affect various parts of the body, potentially leading to health problems if left untreated.

Short-Term Hormonal Contraception: Medications that are hormonal in nature and usually require medical approval. These methods are effective for 3-4 weeks at a time and need replaced every 3-4 weeks. They require the user to use the medication consistently.

Spotting: Very minimal bleeding experience. Can be experienced around ovulation, beginning of menstruation, or end of menstruation. Sometimes blood is only seen when wiping after using the restroom.

Sterilization: Permanent or semi-permanent, sometimes reversible, medical procedure that prevents a person from producing children. For biological females, it typically involves blocking the fallopian tubes or removing the uterus, while for biological men, it usually means cutting or blocking the tubes that carry sperm, all procedures prevent eggs and sperm from meeting.

Sympto-Thermal Method: A way to track changes in the body during the menstrual cycle. It involves observing and recording two main signs: body temperature and cervical mucus, to understand different phases of the cycle and identify patterns in reproductive health.

Tampons: A small, cylindrical product used to absorb menstrual flow. It's inserted into the vagina during menstruation to collect blood before it leaves the body, allowing for comfortable and discreet period management.

The F.I.X. Code: A technology that removes the negative emotional response to a specific memory of a past event or fear so well that when you think about what happened to you; you can't feel that way again. (Can only be done with an Internationally Certified F.I.X. Code Coach) Find our link on page XX of Internationally Certified Coaches.

Tubal Ligation: A surgical procedure involving cutting or blocking the fallopian tubes to prevent eggs from reaching sperm.

Urethra: A tube that carries urine from the bladder out of the body. In females, It's a short tube that ends just above the vaginal opening, while in males, it's longer and runs through the penis.

Urinary System: Is the body's plumbing network that makes and removes urine. It includes the kidneys, which filter blood and produce urine, as well as the bladder, ureters, and urethra, which store and transport urine out of the body.

Uterus: Strong upside-down pear-shaped organ used to carry and grow a baby or babies

Vagina/Vaginal Canal: Is a muscular, hollow tube that extends from the vaginal opening to the cervix. The vagina's muscular walls are lined with mucous membranes, which keep it protected and moist.

Vulva: The external part of the female reproductive system located between the legs and covers the opening to the vagina and other reproductive organs inside the body.

REFERENCE:

Note: all links were retrieved between August and September 2024, they are correct at the time of publication.

* Betts, J. G., Young, K. A., Wise, J. A., Johnson, E., Poe, B., Kruse, D. H., Korol, O., Johnson, J. E., Womble, M., & DeSaix, P. (2022). *Anatomy and physiology.* OpenStax. https://openstax.org/details/books/anatomy-and-physiology
* Strauss, J. & Barbieri, R. (Eds.) (2009). *Yen and Jaffe's Reproductive Endocrinology: Physiology, Pathophysiology, and Clinical Management.* Elsevier Health Sciences.
* Uenoyama, Y., Tsukamura, H. & Maeda, K. (2014), Kisspeptin and puberty. *The Journal of Obstetrics and Gynaecology Research, 40,* 1518-1526. https://doi.org/10.1111/jog.12398
* Brown, J.B. (2011). Types of ovarian activity in women and their significance: the continuum (a reinterpretation of early findings), *Human Reproduction Update, 17*(2), 141-158. https://doi.org/10.1093/humupd/dmq040
* Vigil, P., Lyon, C., Flores, B., Rioseco, H. & Serrano, F. (2017). Ovulation, a sign of health. *The Linacre Quarterly, 84,* 1-13. https://doi.org/10.1080/00243639.2017.1394053
* del Rio, J. & Alliende, I. & Molina, N. & Serrano, F. & Molina, S. & Vigil, P. (2018). Steroid hormones and their action in women's brains: The importance of hormonal balance. *Frontiers in Public Health, 6,* https://doi.org/10.3389/fpubh.2018.00141
* Vigil, P., Ceric, F., Cortés, M.E., & Klaus, H. (2006). Usefulness of monitoring fertility from menarche. *Journal of Pediatric Adolescent Gynaecology, 19*(3), 173-9. https://doi.org/10.1016/j.jpag.2006.02.003
* Vigil, P., del Rio, J., Carrera, B., Aranguiz, C., Rioseco, H. & Cortés Cortés, M. (2016). Influence of sex steroid hormones on the adolescent brain and behavior: An update. *The Linacre Quarterly, 83,* 308-329. https://doi.org/10.1080/00243639.2016.1211863
* Dimitriu, A., & Suni, E. (n.d.). *Teens and Sleep.* https://www.sleepfoundation.org/teens-and-sleep
* Georgopoulos, N., Roupas, N. (2016). Impact of intense physical activity on puberty and reproductive potential of young athletes. In: Vaamonde, D., du Plessis, S., Agarwal, A. (Eds.) *Exercise and human reproduction.* Springer. https://doi.org/10.1007/978-1-4939-3402-7_15
* Klump, K.L., Keel, P.K., Sisk, C., & Burt, S.A. (2010). Preliminary evidence that estradiol moderates genetic influences on disordered

eating attitudes and behaviors during puberty. *Psychological Medicine, 40*, 1745–53. https://10.1017/S0033291709992236

• Vigil, P., Meléndez, J. & Petkovic, G. & del Rio, J. (2022). The importance of estradiol for body weight regulation in women. *Frontiers in Endocrinology*, 13, https://doi.org/10.3389/fendo.2022.951186

• https://publications.aap.org/pediatrics/article/118/5/2245/69874/Menstruation-in-Girls-and-Adolescents-Using-the?autologincheck=redirected

• *Home*. FEMM Health. (2024, August 19). http://www.femmhealth.org/

• *Mjohnson*. Creighton Model. (2023, November 30). https://creightonmodel.com/

• Washburn, S. (2019). *The Revolution Will Be Bloody*.

• Inchauspé, J. (2022). *Glucose revolution: The life-changing power of balancing your blood sugar*. Simon & Schuster Audio.

• https://www.verywellhealth.com/contraceptive-injections-906874

• https://www.mirena-us.com/about-mirena/how-does-mirena-work

• https://www.plannedparenthood.org/learn/birth-control/diaphragm/how-do-i-use-a-diaphragm

• https://my.clevelandclinic.org/health/articles/17979-cervical-cap

Periods are designed to be painfree.

- - - *Heather Allmendinger*

Heather Allmendinger

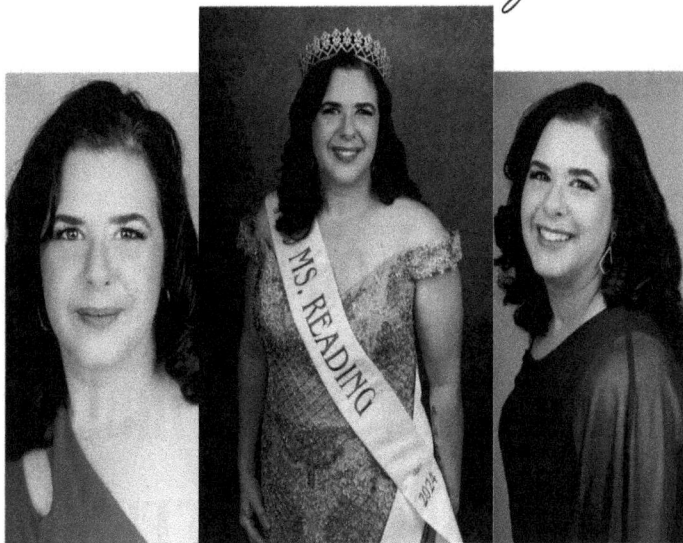

About

Heather, a triple-certified health coach, speaker, and celebrated author, is a recognized pioneer in women's health. She is the Founder of Vivydus, The Full of Life Company, and was a 2024 Business Woman of the Year nominee. As host of the internationally acclaimed Embracing Flow podcast, Heather bridges science and practicality to educate biological female athletes and high achievers on the profound connection between menstrual cycles, performance, and moon phases. Representing her mission as United States of America's Ms. Reading 2024 and Ms. Berks County 2025, she challenges societal norms with humor, honesty, and expertise, empowering women to optimize their well-being and performance from puberty to menopause and beyond.

When You Change The Way You Think, The Things You Think About Change!

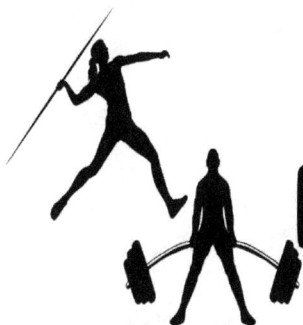

MEET BARB V

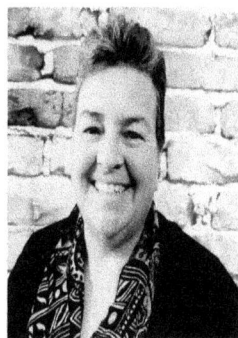

While Barb's career has earned her recognition as an International Gold Medalist with the American Flag and National Anthem raised in her honor across three continents, her true passion lies in helping others achieve their dreams. Starting with her first entrepreneurial venture at age six, she discovered her gift for combining athletic excellence with business innovation to create win-win opportunities for everyone.

This mission became clear upon her college graduation, where she had raised over a million dollars in fundraising support for the teams, schools, clubs and organizations she was a member of during her school years. Today, that same drive fuels her work as an award-winning athletic, personal development, and business coach, where she has dedicated herself to ensuring no athlete has to choose between pursuing their sport and financial stability.

Sharing her strategies and insights with over 300,000 people across 67 countries, Barb has witnessed firsthand how combining the right athletic mindset with business acumen can transform lives. Her international bestselling books serve as roadmaps for athletes, coaches, parents, teams and programs seeking to excel both in their sport and in creating sustainable success. Barb's unique coaching methodology helps countless athletes secure life-changing scholarships and sponsorships, while her company has a specifically designed pathway for post-collegiate athletes to generate the income needed to live, train, and compete on their own terms.

What sets Barb's approach apart is her deep understanding of how to dominate the athlete's journey—because she's still living it. As an active competitor herself, she intimately knows the challenges of balancing athletic pursuits with business development. This firsthand experience drives her to help clients eliminate performance roadblocks, master their mindset, and build successful enterprises that support their athletic dreams.

Through her guidance, athletes aren't just winning medals—they're building legacies. Teams aren't just achieving goals—they're creating sustainable success stories. And coaches aren't just developing programs—they're transforming lives. Every day, Barb's greatest joy comes from seeing her clients break through their perceived limitations and realize possibilities they never imagined existed.

Follow Barb on LinkedIn and Amazon or via her website at BarbV.Fun When you get to know her, you know she doesn't do anything unless it's FUN!

195

Connect with

Barb V

✉ XXStrong@Email.com

📞 +1 918-928-9987

🌐 www.BarbV.Fun

📷 @XXStrong.Life

in /in/XXStrong

in /in/barb-v-81497547/

Connect with

Heather Allmendinger

✉ Heather@Vivydus.com

☎ +1 484-648-0252

🌐 www.Vivydus.com

📷 @vivydus

f fb.com/hmallmendinger

in /in/hmallmendinger

www.ingramcontent.com/pod-product-compliance
Lightning Source LLC
Chambersburg PA
CBHW050118280326
41933CB00010B/1147